PRACTICAL MED

中譯實用醫學

CW00369155

To all those who have taught us:
our teachers, students and most of all, our patients

A HANDBOOK OF

PRACTICAL MEDICAL TERMS
(ENGLISH CHINESE)

中譯實用醫學詞匯

Fourth Edition

William I. Wei 韋霖

MBBS, MS, FRCS, FRCSE, FRACS (Hon),
FHKAM (Surg), FHKAM (ORL)

Stephen W.K. Cheng 鄭永強

MBBS, MS, FRCSE, FACS, FHKAM (Surg)

Anthony Ng 吳崇文

MD, MPH, FRCSE

香港大學出版社
HONG KONG UNIVERSITY PRESS

Hong Kong University Press
The University of Hong Kong
Pokfulam Road
Hong Kong
www.hkupress.org

First edition 1984
Second edition 1989
Third edition 1998
Fourth edition first published 2008; reprinted 2010, 2012, 2014

ISBN 978-962-209-952-4

British Library Cataloguing-in-Publication Data
A catalogue record for this book is available from the British Library.

10 9 8 7 6 5 4

Printed and bound by Livex Ltd., in Hong Kong, China

Contents

Foreword to the Fourth Edition

Practising medicine requires developing a trusting relationship with patients. The ability to understand patients' expectations, and to explain diagnoses and treatments in a way they can comprehend are essential skills for all medical practitioners.

The popular, well-written, and comprehensive English-Chinese *Handbook of Practical Medical Terms* has benefited generations of medical practitioners, from medical students, nurses to experienced doctors. It has been most useful as a handy reference for those practitioners whose first language may not be English or those who wish to know the current Chinese nomenclature of a well known medical term.

The current edition has retained the characteristics of the previous editions, as a quick reference on relevant topics, but it has also incorporated newer medical terms that accompany the advance of medical technology. It remains an indispensable guide to the medical profession, and offers excellent value in terms of content, size and efficient reference.

Dr the Honourable York CHOW Yat-ngok
Secretary for Food and Health
Hong Kong SAR

Preface to the Fourth Edition

Never before has the need to communicate been greater in this day of true multinational collaboration. Doctors in Hong Kong are blessed with exposure to medical knowledge in English and Chinese. On a daily basis we speak to patients and their relatives, participate in academic meetings and write to colleagues, and make new alliances in research in these two languages. As we grew used to Chinese medical terms and became more comfortable in general exchanges over the last decades, new challenges arise as our practices also evolve. With the advancement of technology, we witnessed a rapid change in the treatment options of our patients across all specialties, and new medical terms are created while old names and procedures became obsolete. An expansion of our medical vocabulary calls for an up-to-date, practical guide. This is particularly relevant in view of the increasing interaction between doctors across the border in recent years

A Handbook of Practical Medical Terms (English-Chinese) has been with us for more than two decades. For some, it has been a companion throughout their entire medical career. The book has become the definitive guide, produced by local practising physicians, to English-Chinese medical translation in Hong Kong. This latest edition has been extensively revised by recognized experts in their fields, and is presented in a user-friendly, clearly classified format under different systems and specialties. It is our wish that it will continue to appeal to medical students, allied health providers, nurses, doctors, and patients alike.

We would like to thank all those who have contributed to this fourth edition, without their devoted efforts, this would not be possible.

William I. Wei
Stephen W. K. Cheng
Anthony Ng
June 2008
Hong Kong

Preface to the First Edition

This handbook is written with the Hong Kong medical community in mind. For some time, a communication gap has existed between patients and clinical staff. This gap has widened even more now that treating patients has become more of a science than an art.

The lack of a direct doctor/patient relationship in the public system of health care is an important contributing factor to this gap. The main reason for poor communications is language. Medical students are taught in English. As a result, students and graduates alike all find it difficult to translate their medical knowledge into Chinese — the language most patients can understand and relate to.

As the community becomes more educated, they will demand to know more than just 抽血, 做手術. Better communications not only make for improved relationships and patient care, but also offer a golden opportunity to educate patients about their bodies, in health and in sickness.

This handbook is complied by surgeons — the 'action arm' of the medical profession — who see the vital need to bridge the language gap. The aim is to improve clinican/patient communication. It is not designed for inter-professional communication, where English remains a satisfactory medium. It is intended that it will be studied rather than be used as a reference dictionary, of which many good ones are available.

The reader, whether a student going through a rotation or a practitioner in a specialty, can refer to the respective section easily and quickly, and will be able to master the vocabulary necessary to communicate with the patient.

There are terms which patients will find difficult to understand and which will need further clarification. The degree of comprehension depends upon the level of education of the patients.

It is inevitable that there will be gaps in the handbook. In determining which terms to be included, a practical approach was adopted, the various sections were sent to practising clinicans in the respective fields for verification. Language experts from the Chinese University of Hong Kong were also consulted and difficult translations were only adopted after careful consideration.

The responsibility of the final editing rests with the authors.

We hope that we have made a start in improving 'patient care and communication'.

A. Ng
W.I. Wei
August 1984
Hong Kong

Acknowledgements

We acknowledge the help of the following, in reviewing the various sections of this handbook:

Cheng LC	Chief of Service, Cardiothoracic Surgical Unit, The Grantham Hospital
Kwong, Ava	Associate Consultant, Division of Breast Surgery, Department of Surgery University of Hong Kong Medical Centre
Fang, David	Consultant Orthopaedic Surgeon, St. Paul's Hospital
Ho SL	Professor, Division of Neurology, Department of Medicine, University of Hong Kong Medical Centre
Kung, Annie	Professor, Division of Endocrinology, Department of Medicine, University of Hong Kong Medical Centre
Kwok, Irene	Senior Speech Therapist, Department of ENT, Queen Elizabeth Hospital
Lai CF	Consultant Dermatologist, Hong Kong Sanatorium & Hospital

Lai CL	Professor, Division of Gasteroenterology, Department of Medicine, University of Hong Kong Medical Centre
Lam WK	Professor, Division of Pulmonary Medicine, Department of Medicine, University of Hong Kong Medical Centre
Liang, Raymond	Professor, Division of Haematology/Oncology, Department of Medicine, University of Hong Kong Medical Centre
Li, Walton	Consultant Ophthalmologist, Hong Kong Sanatorium and Hospital
Tang SW	Professor, Department of Psychiatry, University of Hong Kong Medical Centre
Tang WK, Grace	Professor, Department of Obstetrics & Gynaecology, University of Hong Kong Medical Centre
Tong CK, Antonio	Consultant, Senior Dental Officer, Department of Maxillofacial Surgery, Queen Mary Hospital
Wong KK	Consultant Urologist, Hong Kong Sanatorium & Hospital
Yu HC	Chief of Service, Department of ENT, Queen Elizabeth Hospital

1 General 一般通用

abrasion 擦傷

abscess 膿腫 (瘡)

acquired 後天性

acquired immunodeficiency
  syndrome (AIDS)
  後天性免疫缺乏綜合症
  (愛滋病)

acute 急性

addiction 上癮

adenoma 腺瘤

adhesion 黏連

adrenergic 腎上激素性

aggravating factor 惡化因素

agitated 激動 (不安定)

agonist 催動素

airway 呼吸道，空氣通道

albumin 清蛋白

allergy 變態反應 (過敏症)

alleviating factor 緩和因素

allograft 同種移植

anaesthesia, anesthesia
  麻醉，麻醉科

anaesthesiology/
  anaesthesiologist
  麻醉科/麻醉科醫生

analgesic 止痛藥

anaplastic 退變性，反樸性

anatomy/anatomist
  解剖學/解剖學家

anorexia 厭食 (無胃口)

antagonist 反動素

anterior 前

antibiotic 抗菌素 (抗生素)

antihelminthic 杜蟲藥

antihistamine
　抗組織胺藥 (抗敏感藥)

anti-inflammatory drug
　消炎藥

antileprosy drug 痲瘋藥

antimalarial drug 防瘧藥

antineoplastic drug 抗癌藥

antipyretic drug 退熱藥

antiseptic 抗菌藥 (消毒劑)

antituberculous drug
　抗結核菌藥

appendage 附器

arterial blood gas 動脈血氣壓

atresia 閉鎖

atrophy 萎縮

auscultation 聽診

autoantibody 自身抗體

autograft 自體移植

autonomic nervous system
　自主神經系統

autonomic nervous system,
　parasympathetic
　副交感自主神經系統

autonomic nervous system,
　sympathetic
　交感自主神經系統

bacteria 細菌

basal metabolic rate (BMR)
　基本新陳代謝率

benign 良性

bilateral 兩側

biochemistry/biochemist
　生 (物) 化學/生化學家

bionics 生機電子 (仿生學)

biopsy 活組織檢驗

blood bank 血庫

blood pressure 血壓

blood pressure, diastolic
　心舒血壓

blood pressure, systolic
　心縮血壓

blood transfusion 輸血

blunt 鈍

body build 體形

body weight 體重

buffer 中和

cachexia 衰弱

calcification 鈣化

calcium 鈣

carbohydrate 碳水化合物

carbon dioxide 二氧化碳

carbon monoxide 一氧化碳

carcinoma 癌

cardiology/cardiologist
心臟科/心臟醫生

caseation 乾酪化

catabolism 分解性代謝

catheter 導管

cautery 燒灼術

cell 細胞

cell cytoplasm 細胞體漿

cell division 細胞分裂

cell membrane 細胞膜

cell nucleoli 細胞核仁

cell nucleus 細胞核

cellulitis 蜂組織炎

central nervous system
中樞神經系統

certificate 證明

chemotherapy 藥物療法

chest medicine/chest physician
胸肺科/胸肺醫生

chills 寒戰

chloride 氯化物

cholesterol 膽固醇

chromatography 色素分離法

chromosome 染色體

chronic 慢性，慣性

cold, common 傷風，感冒

collapse 虛脫

coma 昏迷

complaint 陳訴，訴苦

complaint, chief 主訴

complication 併發病

condition 情況

condition, critical 情況危殆

condition, deteriorating
情況惡化

condition, fair 情況普通

condition, improving 情況轉佳

condition, labile 情況不穩

condition, poor 情況欠佳

condition, satisfactory
情況滿意

condom 避孕套（安全套）

confused 神智混亂

congenital 先天性

conscious 神智清醒

consent, informed 知會同意

consent form 意願書（同意書）

constitution 體質

consultant 主管醫生
（顧問醫生）

consultation 會診

contagious 接觸傳染

contusion 撞傷（挫傷）

cream 軟膏 (霜)

criteria 準則

cross match 血互配

cryosurgery 冷烙療法

crystal 結晶

cyanosis 發紫，發紺

cycle 周期，循環

cyst 水囊，囊腫

cytology 細胞檢驗

cytology/cytologist
　細胞學/細胞學家

debridement 清創術

decompression 減壓 (解壓)

degeneration 退化

dehydration 脫水，失水

dermatology/dermatologist
　皮膚科/皮膚醫生

dermoid cyst 皮纖維水囊

desmoid tumour 硬纖維瘤

deterioration 惡化

diagnosis 診斷

diagnosis, clinical 臨床診斷

diagnosis, differential
　鑑別診斷

diarrhoea, diarrhea
　腹瀉 (肚痾)

diathermy 透熱燒灼術

dietetics/dietitian, dietician
　營養學/營養學專家

differentiation 分化

differentiated, poorly
　低度分化

differentiated, well 高度分化

discharge 排出物

discharge, purulent
　膿狀排出物

discharge, serosanguineous
　血水性排出物

discharge, serous 水性排出物

disease 病，病症

disinfectant 消毒劑

distress 危急

dominant 顯性

donor 捐贈者

dorsal 背

dose, dosage 劑量

drain 引流

drug 藥物

drug absorption 藥吸收

drug action 藥功能

drug distribution 劑量分佈

dysplasia 增殖不良

dystrophy 增長不良

electrolyte 電游子 (電解質)

electrophoresis 電游子透析法

emaciated 消瘦

endocrinology 內分泌學/
內分泌專家

endocrinology/endocrinologist
內分泌科/內分泌專家

endothelium 內皮

enzyme 酶 (酵素)

epithelium 上皮

erosion 腐蝕 (糜爛)

essential 自發性 (e.g. essential
hypertension) 必需
(e.g. essential amino acid)

essential, non- 必要 (需) 的/
非必要 (需) 的

evaluation 評估

exacerbation 惡化

excision 割除

excrete 排泄

exploratory 探查

extracellular 細胞外

extracellular fluid space
細胞外水空間

exudate 滲出物

failure, cardiac 心機能衰竭

failure, hepatic 肝機能衰竭

failure, renal 腎機能衰竭

failure, respiratory
呼吸機能衰竭

family history 家庭病歷

family physician 家庭醫生

fascia 筋膜

fat 脂肪，肥胖

febrile 發熱 (發燒)

feeling tired 疲倦

feeling weak 虛弱

fever 發熱 (發燒)

fever, high 高熱

fever, low grade 微熱

fever, swinging 反覆性發熱

fibre 纖維

fibrous 纖維的

fistula 瘻，瘻管

fixation 固定，固定法

flu like illness 感冒狀病症

foreign body 異物

friable 易破碎

frozen section 冰凍切片檢驗

fungate 蕈狀潰爛

fungus 霉菌

gangrene 壞疽，壞死

gastroenterology/
gastroenterologist
腸胃科/腸胃醫生

general check up 全身檢查

general practice/general practitioner 全科醫生

general surgery/general surgeon 綜合外科/綜合外科醫生

genetics/geneticist 遺傳學/遺傳學家

gland 腺

glucose 葡萄糖

glycosuria 糖尿

gonococcus 淋球菌

graft 移植，移植物

graft, artificial 人工移植

gram 克

gram, kilo- 千克(公斤)

gram, micro- 微克

gram, milli- 毫克

granulation tissue 肉芽組織

gynaecology/gynaecologist 婦科/婦科醫生

haemangioma 血管瘤

hamartoma 缺陷瘤

hereditary 遺傳

histology/histologist 細胞組織學/細胞組織學家

history 病歷

homeostasis 體內環境恆定

homograft 同種移植

hospital course 住院過程

human immunodeficiency virus (HIV) 破壞免疫病毒(愛滋病毒)

hyperaemia 充血

hyperplasia 增殖

hypersensitivity 過敏性

hypertrophy 增大，肥大

hypnotic 安眠藥

hypoplasia 增殖不良

icterus (jaundice) 黃疸

immunity 免疫性

immunity, acquired 後天免疫性

immunity, natural 先天免疫性

immunization 免疫法

immunology/immunologist 免疫學/免疫學家

immunosuppression 免疫壓制

immunotherapy 免疫療法

infarction 梗塞敗壞

infection 感染，傳染

infectious disease 傳染病

inferior 下，在下

infiltration 浸潤

inflammation 炎，發炎

injection 注射

injection, intra-arterial
動脈注射

injection, intra-articular
關節內注射

injection, intracardiac
心內注射

injection, intramuscular
肌內注射

injection, intra-osseous
骨內注射

injection, intrapleural
胸膜內注射

injection, intrathecal
椎管內注射

injection, intravenous
靜脈注射

injection, subcutaneous
皮下注射

injury 損傷

inoperable 不能切除

inspection 望診

intensity 強度

intensive care unit (ICU)
深切治療部

intern 實習醫生

internal medicine/internist
內科/內科醫生

intoxication 中毒 (醉酒)

intracellular 細胞內

intracellular fluid space
細胞內水空間

irregular 不規則

irritable 容易激動

ischaemia 缺血

isograft 卵雙生子移植

isolation 隔離

jaundice (icterus) 黃疸

keratin 角質素

ketone 酮體

laboratory 化驗室，實驗室

laboratory, biochemical
生物化學化驗室

laboratory, histopathology
組織病理化驗室

laboratory, microbiology
微生 (物) 化驗室

laboratory, serological
血清化驗室

laceration 裂傷

latent 潛伏性

lateral 外側

lecturer 講師

lecturer, senior 高級講師

lesion 損傷

lethal 致命

lethargic 無精打采，懶散

life expectancy 預期壽命

liposuction 脂肪抽除術

litre 公升

litre, micro 微升

litre, milli 毫升

lobe 葉

lotion 外敷液 (洗劑)

lump 硬塊

lymphangioma 淋巴管瘤

magnesium 鎂

malaise 不適

malignant 惡性

management 處理

management, aggressive
　積極處理

management, conservative
　保守處理

mass 腫塊

meatus 道，口

medial 內側

medical officer 醫官

medical officer, senior
　高級醫官

meiosis 減數細胞分裂

metabolism 新陳代謝 (代謝)

metabolism, aerobic
　需氧新陳代謝

metabolism, anaerobic
　缺氧新陳代謝

metastasis 癌轉移，癌擴散

metre 米 (公尺)

metre, centi- 厘米

metre, kilo- 千米

metre, micro- 微米

metre, milli- 毫米

microscope 顯微鏡

microscopy 顯微檢驗

microscopy, electron
　電子顯微鏡檢查

midwifery/midwife
　助產/助產士

mild 溫和，適度

miosis 瞳孔縮少

mitosis 絲狀細胞分裂

moribund 垂死

mortuary 停屍室，殮房

mucosa 黏膜

nausea 作嘔，作悶

necrotic 壞死

neoplasia, neoplasm 癌

nervous 神經緊張

neurological surgery
neurosurgeon 神經系統外科/
神經系統外科醫生

neurology/neurologist
神經病學/神經病學醫生

nucleic acid 核酸

numbness 麻木

obese 肥胖

obstetrics/obstetrician
產科/產科醫生

occupational disease 職業病

occupational therapy 職業療法

oedema, cerebral 腦水腫

oedema, edema 水腫

oedema, pedal 腳水腫

oedema, pulmonary 肺水腫

ointment 軟膏

operating room, operating
theatre 手術室

operation 手術

ophthalmology/
ophthalmologist
眼科/眼科醫生

oral surgery/oral surgeon
口腔外科/口腔外科醫生

orthopaedics 矯形 (外科)

orthopaedic surgery/
orthopaedic surgeon
骨科/骨科醫生

otolaryngology/
otolaryngologist
耳鼻喉科/耳鼻喉科醫生

outpatient department 門診部

oxygen 氧氣

paediatric surgery/paediatric
surgeon
小兒外科/小兒外科醫生

paediatrics/paediatrician
兒科/兒科醫生

pain 痛

pain, abdominal 腹痛，肚痛

pain, burning 灼痛

pain, colicky 絞痛

pain, constant 持續痛

pain, diffuse 分散性痛，
非局部痛

pain, dull 鈍痛

pain, generalized 全面性痛

pain, intermittent 間歇性痛

pain, localized 局部性痛

pain, mild 輕微痛

pain, radiating 擴散痛

pain, referred 相關性痛

pain, severe 劇痛

pain, sharp 尖 (銳) 痛

palliative 姑息

pallor 蒼白

palpation 觸症

palsy 癱瘓

papilla 乳頭狀突起

papilloma 乳頭狀瘤

paraesthesia 異常感覺

parasite 寄生蟲

paroxysmal 陣發性

past history 以往病歷

pathogenesis 病因

pathology/pathologist
  病理學/病理學醫生

percussion 叩診

percutaneous 透皮穿刺

perforation 穿破

pharmacology/pharmacologist
  藥理學/藥理學家

pharmacy/pharmacist
  藥房，藥劑學/藥劑師

physical examination 人體檢驗

physiology/physiologist
  生理學/生理學家

physiotherapy/physiotherapist
  物理治療/物理治療師

placebo 對照測試

placebo effect 代設藥效用

plasma 血漿

plastic surgery/plastic surgeon
  整形外科/整形外科醫生

pneumococcus 肺炎球菌

poisoning 中毒

polyp 息肉

post-operative care 術後照顧

posterior 後

potassium 鉀

pre-operative evaluation
  術前估計

precipitating factor 促成因素

present illness 現病歷

pressure 壓力

pressure, blood 血壓

pressure, osmotic 滲透壓

primary 原發，第一期

professor 教授

prognosis 預期後果

prolapse 脫垂

prophylaxis 預防

protein 蛋白質

proteinuria 蛋白尿

psychiatry/psychiatrist
  精神病學/精神病學醫生

pulse 脈搏

purulent 膿性

qualitative 質

quantitative 量

radiography/radiographer
放射性攝影術/放射性影師

radio-immunoassay
放射免疫分析

radiology/radiologist
放射學/放射學醫生

radioresistant 放射抗拒

radiosensitive 放射感應

radiotherapy 放射治療

reaction 反應

recapse 再發

recessive 隱性

recipient 接受者

recovery 復元

recurrent 復發

regress 退化

regular 有規則

relapse 再發

respiration 呼吸

restless 不安

retention 滯留

retraction 回縮

retroperitoneal fibrosis
腹膜後纖維化

retroperitoneal haematoma
腹膜後血腫

review of systems 系統檢查

rigid 僵硬

rupture 破裂

screen 甄別

secondary 繼發 (第二期)

secrete 分泌

secretion 分泌物

sedative 鎮靜劑

semicomatose 半昏迷

semiconscious 半清醒

septicaemia, septicemia 血中毒

sequelae 後遺症

serous 漿液性

severe 沉重，嚴重

sex-linked heredity
性別相連遺傳

shock 休克，震驚

sick leave 病假

side effect 副作用

sign 病徵

sinus 竇

social history 個人生活史

sodium 鈉

somatic 軀體

spasm 痙攣 (抽筋)

specialty/specialist
專科/專科醫生

specific gravity 比重

sphincter 括約肌

sphincter tone 括約肌張力

sphygmomanometer 血壓計

squamous 鱗狀

staphylococcus 葡萄球菌

stasis 積滯

state of consciousness 清醒狀態

state of health 健康狀態

stethoscope 聽診器 (聽診)

streptococcus 鏈球菌

stupor 僵呆，神智不清

subacute 亞急性

subluxation 半脫位

superior 上

suppurative 化膿

surgery/surgeon 外科/外科醫生

survival rate 生存率

survival rate, five year 五年生存率

survival rate, median 中線生存率

suture 縫合，縫綫

symptom 症狀

syndrome 綜合症，綜合徵狀

system 系統

tachypnoea 氣促，呼吸急促

telangiectasis 微絲血管擴張

temperature 體溫

tenderness 壓痛

tenderness, rebound 反彈痛

tertiary 第三期，後期

therapeutics 治療法

therapy (see treatment) 治療

tissue 組織

toxic 有毒

toxic effect 毒性效果

toxicology/toxicologist 毒理學/毒理學家

transitional epithelium 過渡性上皮

trauma 外傷，創傷

treatment 治療，療法

treatment, conservative 保守治療

treatment, cytotoxic 抗細胞治療

treatment, general 一般治療

treatment, hormonal 激素治療

treatment, local 局部治療

treatment, palliative 姑息治療

treatment, radiation 放射治療

treatment, specific 特殊治療

treatment, symptomatic
症狀治療

triglyceride 三酸甘油脂

tumour 腫瘤 (癌)

ulcer 潰瘍

unconscious 昏迷 (不省人事)

undifferentiated 未分化

urological surgery/urological
surgeon
泌尿外科/泌尿系統外科醫生

vaccine 疫苗

valve 瓣

vascular pedicle 血管蒂

vascular surgery/vascular
surgeon
血管外科/血管外科醫生

vasoconstriction 血管收縮

venipuncture
靜脈穿刺術 (抽血)

virus 過濾性病菌 (病毒)

visceral 臟腑，內臟

vitamin 維生素

vomit 嘔吐

ward 病房

wart 疣

weak 虛弱

wheeze 哮鳴

withdrawal symptom 脫癮病狀

xenograft 異種移植

2 Eye 眼

abrasion 擦傷

accommodation 調節力，調整

amblyopia 弱視

anisocoria 瞳孔不等

aphakia 無晶狀體

aqueous humour
　（水狀液）眼房水

astigmatism 散光

blepharitis 瞼邊緣炎

blepharon 瞼邊緣

canthus 眼角

cataract 白內障 (起膜)

cataract, junvenile 幼年白內障

cataract, mature 成熟白內障

cataract, senile 老年白內障

cataract, traumatic
　外傷性白內障

chalazion (internal
　hordeolum) 內瞼腺炎

chamber, anterior 眼前房

chamber, posterior 眼後房

choroid 脈胳膜

cilia 纖毛

ciliary body 纖毛體

colour blindness 色弱

conjunctiva 眼結膜

contact lens 接觸鏡片
　（隱形眼鏡）

contusion / eye contusion
眼挫傷

cornea 眼角膜

cornea abrasion 眼角膜擦損

cornea transplant 眼角膜移植

cornea ulcer 角膜潰瘍

cryosurgery 冷凍手術

cycloplegia 睫狀肌麻痹

dacryocystitis, chronic
慢性淚囊炎

dark adaptation 暗適應

dendritic ulcer 樹枝狀潰瘍

diplopia 複視 (疊影)

disc, optic 視盤

discharge 排泌

ectropion 眼瞼外翻

electroretinography
視網膜電圖

enophthalmos 眼球陷入

entropion 眼瞼內翻

enucleation 眼球摘除術

epicanthus 內眥贅皮

epiphora 淚溢 (淚水過多)

exophthalmos 眼球突出 (突眼)

extra-ocular movement
眼外肌動作

eye drops 眼藥水

eye pad 眼墊

eyeball 眼球

eyebrow 眼眉

eyelash 眼睫毛

eyelid 眼蓋

fornix 穹窿

fracture, blow out 眼眶爆裂

fundus 眼底

glaucoma 青光眼
(綠內障或眼壓增高)

glaucoma, narrow angle
窄角青光眼

glaucoma, open angle
闊角青光眼

globe 眼球

haemorrhage, punctate
點狀出血

haemorrhage, subconjunctival
結膜下出血

hemianopia 偏盲

hordeolum 瞼腺炎

hypermetropia (far
sightedness) 遠視

hyphema 眼前房積血

icterus 黃疸

infraorbital 眶下

injection, capillary
微絲血管充血

intra-ocular foreign body
眼內異物

intra-ocular pressure 眼內壓

iridectomy 虹膜切除術

iridocyclitis 虹膜睫狀體炎

iris 虹膜

iritis 虹膜炎

irrigation 冲洗

keratitis 角膜炎

keratitis, herpetic 疱疹角膜炎

keratoconjunctivitis
角膜結膜炎

keratomalacia 角膜軟化

lacrimal duct 淚管

lacrimal gland 淚腺

lacrimal sac 淚囊

lacrimation 流淚

laser 激光

**LASIK (laser in-situ
keratomileusis)**
角膜切割激光矯視手術

lens 晶狀體

lenticular opacity 晶狀體混濁

leucoma 角膜白斑

lid lag 眼蓋活動遲鈍

light reflex 光反射

limbus 眼緣 (角鞏膜交界)

macula 黃斑點 (角膜斑)

meibomian cyst 瞼板腺囊腫

micro aneurysm 微絲動脈瘤

miotic 縮瞳藥

mydriatic 擴瞳藥

myopia (short-sightedness)
近視

nebula 角膜雲翳

neovascularization 血管新生

nerve, abducent 外展神經

nerve, oculomotor 動眼神經

nerve, optic 視神經

nerve, trochlear 滑輪神經

night blindness 夜盲

nystagmus 眼球震顫

ointment 軟膏

ophthalmodynamometry
眼動脈血壓計

ophthalmology/
ophthalmologist
眼科/眼科醫生

ophthalmoplegia 眼肌麻痺

ophthalmoscope 眼窺鏡

optic atrophy 視神經衰萎

optic nerve 視神經

optic neuritis 視神經炎

optician 眼鏡技師

orbit 眼眶

palpebra 眼瞼

palpebral conjunctiva
眼瞼結膜

palpebral oedema 眼瞼浮腫

papilloedema, papilledema
視神經乳頭體水腫

photocoagulation 激光凝固

photophobia 畏光

presbyopia 老花 (遠視)

pterygium 翼狀胬肉

ptosis 眼上蓋下垂

pupil 瞳孔

refraction 折光 (驗眼)

refractive 屈光

refractive power 屈光力

rupture 破裂

retina 視網膜

retinal detachment
視網膜脫落

retinal artery/vein
視網動/靜脈

retinoblastoma
視網膜胚細胞癌

retinopathy 視網膜病變

retinopathy, diabetic
糖尿性視網膜病變

retinopathy, hypertensive
高血壓性視網膜病變

sclera 鞏膜

scotoma 暗點

slit lamp 裂隙燈

strabismus 斜視 (鬥雞眼)

strabismus (convergent
squint) 內斜視

strabismus (divergent squint)
外斜視

stye (external hordeolum)
外瞼腺炎

subconjunctival haemorrhage
結膜下出血

subluxation 半脫症

supraorbital 眼眶上

sympathetic ophthalmia
交感性眼炎

synechia 虹膜黏連

tonometer 眼壓計

tonometry 眼壓測定法

trachoma 沙眼

trichiasis 倒睫毛

ultraviolet light 紫外光

uvea 眼色膜

uveitis 眼色膜炎

vision 視覺

vision, blurred 視覺模糊

visual acuity 視力

visual apparatus 視覺器官

visual field 視野

vitreous humour 玻璃狀體液

xerophthalmia 乾眼病

3

Ear, Nose and Throat
耳，鼻，喉

acoustic neuroma 聽覺神經瘤

adenoid 增殖腺

adenoidectomy 增殖腺切除術

ala nasi 鼻翼

ameloblastoma
  (adamantinoma)
  釉質母細胞瘤

antehelix 對耳輪

agraphia (dysgrapahia) 失寫症

alaryngeal speech 無喉發聲

alexia (dyslexia) 失讀症

aphasia (dysphasia) 失語症

apraxia (dyspraxia) 失用症

articulation disorder 構音異常

artificial larynx 人造喉頭

arytenoid 杓狀輭骨

audiogram 聽力測驗圖

audiometry 聽力測驗法

auditory training 聽能訓練

aural rehabilitation 聽能復康

auricle 耳廓

autism 自閉症

babbling 牙牙學語

bilingualism 雙重語言

biopsy 活組織檢驗

branchia 鰓

branchial abscess 鰓膿腫

branchial cyst 鰓囊

branchial fistula 鰓瘻管

buccal mucosa 頰粘膜

buccal speech 頰語

Caldwell Luc operation
  領竇手術 (領竇黏膜清除術)

carcinoma, alveolus 牙槽癌

carcinoma, larynx 喉癌

carcinoma, tongue 舌癌

carcinoma, tonsillar fossa
  扁桃窩癌

carotid body tumour
  頸動脈體瘤

cartilage 軟骨

catarrh 黏膜炎

cerumen 耳蠟

cheek 面頰

cheilosis 唇乾裂

choanal atresia 鼻後孔閉鎖

cholesteatoma 膽脂瘤

cleft lip 裂唇

cleft palate 裂腭

cochlea 耳蝸

cochlear implant 電子耳蝸

combined resection
  合併切除術

conduction 傳導

conduction, air 空氣傳導

conduction, bone 骨傳導

consonant 聲母

contact ulcer 接觸性潰瘍

cord thickening 聲帶增厚

coryza 鼻炎

cystic hygroma
  水囊狀淋巴管瘤

deafness 聾

decongestant 減充血藥

deviated septum 鼻中隔偏斜

diplophonia 複聲

dizziness 頭暈，頭昏

dysphagia (吞嚥障礙)

dysarthria 吶吃

ear drum 耳膜

ear, external 外耳

ear, inner 內耳

ear lobule 耳珠

echolalia 鸚鵡式學語

edentulous 無牙

electro-laryngeal speech
  電子喉發聲

electronic larynx
  電喉 (電子助講器)

endotracheal tube 氣管內管

epiglottis 會厭

epistaxis 流鼻血

epulis 齦瘤

Eustachian tube
  耳咽管 (歐氏管)

exostosis 外生骨 (骨刺)

facial nerve 面神經

facial nerve palsy 面神經麻痺

fiberoptic endoscopic
  examination of swallowing
  (FEES) 內窺鏡吞嚥檢查

fiberoptic endoscopic
  examination of sensory
  testing (FEEST) 內窺鏡咽喉
  感覺測試

frenulum 繫帶

frequency 頻率

functional aphonia 機能性失聲

functional dysphonia
  機能性發聲障礙

functional endoscopic sinus
  surgery (FESS)
  功能性內窺鏡鼻竇外科

glossitis 舌炎

granuloma 肉芽

grommet 中耳導管

harelip (cleft lip) 裂唇

hearing aids 助聽器

hearing loss 聽覺消失

hearing test 聽覺測驗

helix 耳輪

herpes labialis 唇疱疹

herpes simplex 單純性疱疹

hoarseness 聲嘶

hyoid 舌骨

hypernasality 鼻音過重

hyponasality 鼻音過低

incus 耳砧骨

inhalation method 吸入法

injection method 注入法

intranasal antrostomy
  鼻內鼻竇切開術

intranasal ethmoidectomy
  鼻內篩竇黏膜清除術

language 語言

laryngectomy 喉切除術

laryngitis 喉炎

laryngoscopy 喉鏡檢查

larynx 喉

leucoplakia 白斑

light reflex 光反射

lingual frenulum
  舌繫帶 (腒根)

lip 唇

lip reading 唇讀

malleus 耳錘骨

mandible 下頜骨

mastoid 乳突狀骨

mastoidectomy
乳突狀骨切除術

mastoiditis 乳突狀骨炎

meatus, auditory 聽道口

Meniere's disease 耳病性眩暈

motion sickness
動性眩暈 (暈浪)

mucous membrane 黏膜

mucus 黏液

myringoplasty 耳膜整形術

myringotomy 耳膜割開術

nasal polyp 鼻息肉

nasal polypectomy
鼻息肉切除術

nasal resonance 鼻腔共鳴

nasal septum 鼻中隔

**nasopharyngeal carcinoma
(NPC)** 鼻咽癌

nose 鼻

nostril 鼻孔

obstructive sleep apnoea
阻塞性睡眠呼吸窒息

oesophageal speech 食道語

olfactory 嗅覺

olfactory apparatus 嗅覺器官

oral hygiene 口腔衛生

oral resonance 口腔共鳴

ossicle 耳小骨

ossicle transplant 耳小骨移植

ossiculoplasty 耳小骨整形術

osteoma 骨瘤

osteosclerosis (otosclerosis)
耳小骨硬化

otitis 耳炎

otitis externa 外耳炎

otitis media 中耳炎

**otitis media, acute
suppurative** 急性化膿中耳炎

**otitis media, chronic
suppurative** 慢性化膿中耳炎

otoscope 耳鏡

palate 腭

palate, hard 硬腭

palate, soft 軟腭

papilloma 乳頭狀腫瘤

parotid 腮腺

parotid adenolymphoma
腮腺淋巴瘤

parotid carcinoma 腮腺癌

parotid mixed tumour
腮腺混合性瘤

parotitis 腮腺炎

perichondrial cyst
耳廓輭骨水囊

perichondritis of pinna
耳廓輭骨膜炎

pharyngeal speech 咽語

pharyngitis 咽炎

pharyngoesophageal segment
假聲門

pharynx 咽

pharynx, nasal 鼻咽

pharynx, oral 口咽

phonation 發音

phonctics 音韻學

pinna 耳廓

pitch 音調

pneumatic alaryngeal speech
氣動式咽語

polyp 息肉

polysomnography (sleep
study) 睡眠功能測試

preauricular sinus 耳前竇

pyriform fossa 梨狀窩

radical cervical
lymphadenectomy
頸淋巴組織徹底切除術

radical neck dissection
頸淋巴組織徹底切除術

radiotherapy 放射治療

resonance disorder 共鳴誤差

rhinitis 鼻炎

rhinitis, allergic 敏感性鼻炎

rhinitis, vasomotor
血管神經性鼻炎

rhinoplasty 鼻整形術

rhinorrhoea 流鼻液 (流鼻涕)

salivary gland 唾液腺

salivary gland, parotid
腮唾液腺

salivary gland, sublingual
舌下唾液腺

salivary gland, submandibular
頷下唾液腺

septoplasty 鼻中隔整形術

septum, nasal 鼻中隔

sialoadenitis 唾液腺炎

sinus, paranasal 副鼻竇

sinus, ethmoid 篩竇

sinus, maxillary 上頷竇

sinus, sphenoid 蝶竇

sinusitis 鼻竇炎

smell 嗅覺

spastic dysphonia
痙攣性發聲障礙

speech 言語

speech discrimination
語音聽辨力

speech recognition 語音認知力

speech sound 語音

stapedectomy 耳鐙骨切除術

stapes 耳鐙骨

stomatitis 口腔炎

stuttering/stammering 口吃

taste 味覺

thrush 念珠菌口炎 (鵝口瘡)

thyroglossal cyst 甲狀腺舌囊

thyroglossal duct
　甲狀腺舌導管

tinnitus 耳鳴

tones 聲調

tongue 舌

tongue, base of 舌基

tonsil 扁桃體

tonsillitis 扁桃體炎

tonsil, faucial 腭扁桃體

tonsil, lingual 舌扁桃體

tonsillectomy 扁桃體切除術

total laryngectomy
　全喉切除手術

trachea 氣管

tracheoesophageal speech
　氣管食道語

tracheostomy 氣管造口術

tragus 耳屏

tuning fork 音叉

turbinate (superior, middle,
　inferior) 鼻甲骨 (上、中、下)

tympanic membrane 耳膜

tympanic perforation
　耳膜穿破

tympanometry 耳膜張力測定器

upper respiratory infection
　(URI) 上呼吸道感染

uvula 懸壅 (小舌)

uvulopalatopharyngoplasty
　會厭腭咽形成術

ventricular phonation
　假聲帶發聲

vertigo 眩暈 (天旋地轉)

vestibular function 前庭的機能

vibrissae 鼻毛

videofluroscopic study of
　swallowing (VFSS)
(吞鋇X光造影吞嚥檢查)

vocabulary 字彙

vocal nodule 聲帶小結

vocal paralyses 聲帶攤瘓

vocal polyps 聲帶息肉

vomer 犁骨

vowel 韻母

zygoma 顴骨

Endocrine/Metabolism
內分泌/新陳代謝

ablation 部分切除術

acetone 丙酮

acidosis 血酸中毒

acromegaly 肢端巨大症

Addison's crisis 缺留鈉素危機

Addison's disease 缺留鈉素症

adenocarcinoma 腺癌

adenohypophysis 腦垂體前葉

adenoma 腺瘤

adolescence 青春期

adrenal 腎上腺

adrenal cortex 腎上腺皮層

adrenal cortical trophic hormone (ACTH)
　腎上腺皮質激素

adrenal corticosteroids
　腎上腺皮質素

adrenal medulla 腎上腺髓質

adrenalectomy 腎上腺切除術

adrenaline 腎上腺素

aldosterone 留鈉素

alkalosis 鹼中毒

amine precursor uptake decarboxylase (APUD)
　原氨吸收脫酸酶

amino acid 氨基酸

amyloidosis 澱粉樣變性

angiotensin 血管緊張素

antidiuretic hormone 制尿素

autoantibody 自身抗體

basal metabolic rate (BMR)
基本新陳代謝率

body weight 體重

calciferol 鈣固醇

calcitonin 降鈣素

calcium 鈣

carbohydrate 碳水化合物

carcinoid syndrome
類癌綜合症

central venous catheter
中心靜脈導管

central venous pressure
中心靜脈壓

cholecystokinin 縮膽囊素

cholesterol 膽固醇

Conn's syndrome
留鈉素過多綜合症

constipation 便秘

control 控制，調節

corticosteroid 腎上腺皮質素

cretinism 呆小症

Cushing's disease
腎上腺皮質機能亢進

deficiency 缺乏，不足

dehydration 脫水，失水

diabetes insipidus 尿崩症

diabetes mellitus 糖尿病

diarrhoea, diarrhea
腹瀉 (肚疴)

diet 飲食，節食

dietetics/dietitian, dietician
營養學/營養學家

dwarfism 侏儒病

ectopic 異位的

empty sella syndrome
空碟鞍綜合症

endogenous 內生

enzyme 酶

excess 過度，過多

exophthalmos 眼球凸出

fatigue 疲勞

fatty acid 脂肪酸

feedback 反饋

feminization 女性化

**follicle-stimulating hormone
(FSH)** 卵胞激素

fructose 果糖

galactorrhoea 乳漏

gastric acid analysis 胃酸分析

gastrin 促胃液素

genitalia 生殖器官

genitalia, ambiguous
生殖器官異常

gigantism 畸形巨大症

gland 腺

glucagon 高血糖素

glucocorticoids 激糖素

glucose 葡萄糖

goitre 甲狀腺腫大

goitre, diffuse
彌散性甲狀腺腫大

goitre, endemic
地方性甲狀腺腫大

goitre, multinodular
多結節性甲狀腺腫大

goitre, simple
單純性甲狀腺腫大

goitre, toxic 毒性甲狀腺腫大

gout 痛風

Graves' disease
彌散毒性甲狀腺腫大

growth hormone 生長激素

gynaecomastia 男性乳房腫大

**haemachromatosis,
hemachromatosis**
血色素沉著症

Hashimoto's disease
淋巴性甲狀腺炎

hirsutism 毛髮過多

histamine 組織胺

homeostasis 體內環境恆定

hormone 激素 (內分泌)

hormone, adiponectin 消脂素

hormone, adrenal 腎上腺素

**hormone, adrenal cortical
trophic (ACTH)**
腎上腺皮質激素

**hormone, adrenal
corticosteroids** 腎上腺皮質素

hormone, adrenaline 腎上腺素

hormone, aldosterone 留鈉素

hormone, antidiuretic 制尿素

hormone, cholecystokinin
縮膽囊素

hormone, oestrogen, estrogen
雌激素

**hormone, follicular
stimulating (FSH)** 卵胞激素

hormone, gastrin 促胃液素

hormone, glucagon 高血糖素

hormone, glucocorticoid
激糖素

hormone, gonadotrophin
性腺激素

hormone, growth 生長激素

**hormone, human chorionic
gonadotrophin (HCG)**
胎盤性腺激素

hormone, insulin 胰島素

hormore, leptin 瘦素

hormone, luteinizing (LH) 黃體激素

hormone, melanocyte-stimulating (MSH) 黑細胞激素

hormone, noradrenaline 副腎上腺素

hormone, oxytocin 催產素

hormone, pancreozymin 胰激素

hormone, parathyroid 甲狀旁腺素

hormone, progesterone 孕激素

hormone, prolactin 催乳素

hormone, prostaglandin 前列腺素

hormone, renin 腎素

hormone, secretin 腸促胰液素

hormone, somatotrophin 生長激素

hormone, testosterone 雄激素 (睪丸酮)

hormone, thyroid stimulating (TSH) 甲狀腺激素

hormone, thyroxine 甲狀腺素

hormone, vasoactive intestine 腸血管激素

hormone, vasopressin 加壓素

hormone therapy 激素治療

human chorionic gonadotrophin (HCG) 胎盤性腺激素

hydrocortisone 氫考地松

hyperalimentation (see total parenteral nutrition) 全靜脈營養

hypercalcaemia 血鈣過多

hyperglycaemia 血糖過多

hyperkalaemia 血鉀過多

hypernatraemia 血鈉過多

hyperosmolar 滲透過多

hyperparathyroidism 甲狀旁腺機能過盛

hyperpigmentation 皮膚色素過多

hyperplasia 增殖

hypersecretion 分泌過多

hyperthyroid 甲狀腺機能過盛

hypocalcaemia 血鈣過少

hypoglycaemia 血糖過少

hypokalaemia 血鉀過少

hyponatraemia 血鈉過少

hypoparathyroidism 甲狀旁腺機能減退

hypophysectomy 腦垂體切除術

hypophysis 腦垂體

hyposecretion 分泌不足

hypothalamus 下丘腦

hypothyroid 甲狀腺機能減退

immune response 免疫反應

insulin 胰島素

intravenous nutrition (see total parenteral nutrition) 靜脈營養

ketoacidosis 酮酸中毒

ketone 酮體

lactic acidosis 乳酸中毒

lethargy 無精打采，懶散

libido 性慾

luteinizing hormone (LH) 黃體激素

maltose 麥糖

masculinization 男性化

melanin 黑色素

melanocyte-stimulating hormone (MSH) 黑細胞激素

metabolism 新陳代謝(代謝)

metabolism, aerobic 需氧新陳代謝

metabolism, anaerobic 缺氧新陳代謝

mitochondria 綫粒體

moon face 月狀面形

multiple endocrine neoplasia (MEN I) 多發性內分泌腺瘤一形

multiple endocrine neoplasia (MEN II) 多發性內分泌腺瘤二形

Myasthenia gravis 重症肌無力

myxoedema 黏液性水腫

nervous 神經緊張

neurohypophysis 腦垂體後葉

noradrenaline 副腎上腺素

nutrition 營養

nutrition, intravenous 靜脈營養

nutrition, total parenteral (TPN) 全靜脈營養

obesity 肥胖

oedema, edema 水腫

oestradiol, estradiol 雌素二醇

oestrogen, estrogen 雌激素

oophorectomy 卵巢切除術

optic atrophy 視盤萎縮

orchidectomy 睪丸切除術

osmolality 滲透力度

osmotic diuresis 滲透性利尿

osmotic pressure 滲透壓

osteomalacia 骨軟化

osteoporosis 骨質疏鬆

ovary 卵巢

oxytocin 催產素

palpitation 心悸

pancreas 胰

parathyroid 甲狀旁腺

parathyroid hormone
  甲狀旁腺素

parathyroidectomy
  甲狀旁腺切除術

peptide 蛋白素

phaeochromocytoma
  副神經腺瘤

phospholipid 磷脂

pigmentation 色素沉著

pineal 松果體

pituitary 腦垂體

pituitary fossa 腦垂體窩

polydipsia 多喝

polyphagia 多食

polyuria 多尿

precocious 早熟

primary 原發的，第一期

progesterone 孕激素

prolactin 催乳素

prolactinoma 催乳素瘤

proptosis 凸眼

prostaglandin 前列腺素

protein 蛋白質

puberty 發育期

radioactive iodine 放射性碘

radioactive iodine (RAI)
  uptake 放射性碘吸收

radio-immunoassay
  放射性免疫分析

radiotherapy 放射治療

relaxin 鬆弛素

releasing factor
  促因 (下丘腦分泌)

releasing factor,
  corticotrophin
  腎上腺皮層激素促因

releasing factor, FSH
  卵胞激素促因

releasing factor, GH
  生長激素促因

releasing factor, LH
  黃體激素促因

releasing factor, MSH
  黑細胞激素促因

releasing factor, TSH
甲狀腺激素促因

renin 腎素

retinal exudate 視網膜滲出物

retinal haemorrhage
視網膜出血

retinopathy 視網膜病

rickets 佝僂病 (軟骨病)

scan 掃描

scan, nuclear 放射性素描

scan, thyroid 甲狀腺素描

scan, ultrasound 超音波素描

scurvy 壞血病

secondary 繼發的 (第二期)

secrete, secretion
分泌，分泌物

secretin 腸促胰液素

sella turcica 蝶鞍

serum hormone level
血內分泌度

serum thyroxine level
血甲狀腺素度

sexual characteristic 性特徵

steroid 類固醇

storage 貯藏

stria 紋

subclavian vein puncture
鎖骨下靜脈穿刺

synthesis 合成

testis 睪丸

testosterone 睪丸素 (雄激素)

thymus 胸腺

thyroid 甲狀腺

thyroid crisis
甲狀腺功能亢進危機

thyroid isthmus 甲狀腺峽

thyroid nodule 甲狀腺結節

**thyroid stimulating hormone
(TSH)** 甲狀腺激素

thyroidectomy 甲狀腺切除術

thyroiditis 甲狀腺炎

thyrotoxicosis 甲狀腺毒症

thyrotrophin 促甲狀腺素

thyroxine T$_3$ 三碘甲狀腺素

thyroxine T$_4$ 四碘甲狀腺素

**total parenteral nutrition
(TPN)** 全靜脈營養

transport 輸送

tremor 震顫

triglyceride 甘油三酸酯

truncal obesity 軀體肥胖

uric acid 尿酸

vasoactive intestinal hormone 腸血管激素

vasopressin 加壓素

virilization 男性化

weakness 虛弱

xanthelasma 黃斑瘤

Zollinger-Ellison syndrome 胃酸激素過多綜合症

5 Skin/Breast 皮膚/乳房

a-v malformation 動靜脈變形

abscess 膿疱

acanthosis nigricans 黑棘皮症

acne 暗瘡，青春豆 (痤瘡)

adjuvant therapy 輔藥

AIDS 後天自身免疫系統缺乏症
(愛滋病)

albinism 白化病

alopecia 脫髮，禿

alopecia areata 斑禿 (鬼剃頭)

alopecia totalis 全頭禿

alopecia universalis
全體性脫毛

amyloidosis 澱粉樣變性

angioma 血管瘤

antibiotic 抗菌素 (抗生素)

antihistamine
抗組織胺藥 (抗敏感藥)

antiseptic 抗菌藥 (消毒劑)

atrophy 萎縮

atypical ductal hyperplasia
非典型腺管增生

autoimmune disease
自體免疫病

balanitis 龜頭炎

basal cell carcinoma
基底細胞癌

bedsore 褥瘡

beriberi 腳氣病

blister 水疱

BRCA gene mutation
BRCA 基因突變

breast abscess 乳房膿腫

breast 乳房

breast abscess 乳房膿腫

breast carcinoma, intraductal
管內性乳癌

breast carcinoma, lobular
小葉性乳癌

breast conserving surgery
乳線癌局部切除手術或
保留乳房手術

breast lump 乳房硬塊

bruise 瘀，挫傷

bulla 大疱

burn 灼傷，燒傷

candidiasis 念珠菌病

carbuncle 癰

chancre 梅毒下疳 (硬疳)

chancroid 軟疳

chlamydia 衣原體

chemotherapy 抗癌藥物治療

chicken pox 水痘

chloasma 黃褐斑 (蝴蝶斑)

chilblain 凍瘡

collagen 膠蛋白

collagen disease 膠蛋白病

comedone 粉刺

condyloma acuminatum
尖形濕疣

condyloma lata 扁平濕疣

connective tissue 結締組織

core biopsy
腫瘤核心組織檢查法

corns 椎

corticosteroid 腎上腺皮層素

crack 裂

cream 軟膏 (霜)

crust 痂

dandruff 頭皮屑 (頭皮)

dermabrasion 磨皮手術

dermatitis 皮膚炎

dermatitis, allergic
過敏性皮膚炎

dermatitis, contact
接觸性皮膚炎

dermatitis, exfoliative
剝脫性皮膚炎

dermatitis herpetiformis
疱疹狀皮膚炎

dermatofibroma 皮膚纖維瘤

dermatomyositis 皮肌炎

dermis 真皮

DCIS 原位導管癌

DIEP flap reconstruction
腹下部皮瓣移植術

ductal ectasia 腺管擴張

ductogram 乳管內視鏡

eczema 濕疹

eczema, atopic 異位性濕疹

elastic tissue 彈性纖維

epidermis 表皮

epidermoid cyst 粉瘤

erosion 腐蝕 (糜爛)

erysipelas 丹毒

erythema 紅斑

erythema multiforme
多形性紅斑

erythema nodosum
結節性紅斑

excisional biopsy
割除性活組織檢驗

excoriation 表皮脱落

fat necrosis 脂肪壞死

fibroadenoma 纖維性腺瘤

fibroadenosis 乳腺增生

fibroblast 纖維母細胞

fibrocystic disease
纖維性囊腫病

fibroma 纖維瘤

fibrosis 纖維化

fissure 裂

folliculitis 毛囊炎

frostbite 凍瘡

furuncle 癤

gangrene 壞疽，壞死

German measles 德國痲疹

granulation tissue 肉芽組織

granuloma 肉芽腫

gonococcus infection 淋病

granuloma pyogenicum
化膿性肉芽

gumma 梅毒瘤

gynaecomastia 男性乳房腫大

haemangioma 血管瘤

haemangioma, capillary
微絲血管瘤 (焰色痣)

haemangioma, cavernous
海綿狀血管瘤

haemangioma, strawberry
楊莓狀血管瘤

hair 毛，髮

hair follicle 毛囊

herpes 疱疹

herpes simplex 單純疱疹

herpes zoster, shingles
帶狀疱疹 (生蛇)

histology/histologist
細胞組織學/細胞組織學家

hookwire excision
環狀線切除術

hormone therapy 激素治療

Hutchison's melanotic freckle
黑素雀斑

hyperhidrosis 多汗症

hyperkeratosis 表皮角化病

hypersensitivity reaction
過敏反應

hypertrophy 增大，肥大

ichthyosis 魚鱗癬

impetigo 膿疱病

incision and drainage
(I and D) 切開引流

infection 感染

inflammatry breast cancer
炎性乳腺癌

intertrigo 摺爛 (擦爛)

intraductal papillomatosis
管內乳頭狀瘤病

invasive breast carcinoua
浸潤性乳腺癌

itch 癢

Kaposi's sarcoma 加波氏肉瘤

keloid 瘢痕

keratin 角質素

keratosis 角化病

keratosis, seborrhoeic
皮脂性角化病 (老人痣)

keratosis, senile 老年角化病

lactation 泌乳

lanolin 羊脂

lentigo 色斑

leprosy 痲瘋

leucoplakia 白斑病

lichen planus 扁平苔癬

lipoma 脂肪瘤

liposarcoma 脂肪內癌

lobular 小葉性

lotion 外敷液 (洗劑)

lymphedema 淋巴腫

louse 虱

lupus vulgaris
皮膚結核狼瘡 (尋常狼瘡)

macule 斑疹

mammary dysplasia
乳細胞增殖不良

mammography 乳房 X 光檢查

mammoplasty augmentation
乳房增大整形術 (隆胸術)

mammoplasty reduction
乳房縮小整形術

mammotome 微創乳房切片診
斷系統

mastectomy 乳房切除術

mastectomy, modified radical
改良乳房徹底切除術

mastectomy, radical
乳房徹底切除術

mastectomy, simple
單純乳房切除術

mastitis 乳腺炎

measles 痲疹

medullary carcinoma
乳腺髓樣癌

melanin 黑色素

melanocyte-stimulating
hormone (MSH) 黑細胞激素

melanoma 黑素癌

menopause 閉經 (收經)

menopausal, post- 閉經後

menopausal, pre- 閉經前

microcalifications 乳房內微鈣
化灶

microdochectomy 針刺乳頭吸
取術

milium 酒米

mite 蟎

mole 痣

molluscum contagiosum
傳染性軟疣

molluscum sebaceum
皮脂性軟疣

MRI breast 磁力共振乳腺掃描

naevus 痣

naevus, compound 複合痣

naevus, intradermal 真皮內痣

naevus, junction 真表皮接口痣

naevus, pigmented 色素痣

nail / finger nail / toe nail
甲／指甲／趾甲

neoadjuvant 新輔助治療

neurofibromatosis
多發性神經纖維瘤

nipple 乳頭

nipple discharge 乳頭排出物

oestrogen receptor assay
雌激素受體分析

ointment 油膏

oophorectomy 卵巢切除術

osteo myocutaneous flap
骨肌皮瓣

onychomycosis 甲癬 (灰甲)

Paget's disease of nipple
乳頭癌變病

papule 丘疹

paste 糊

patch test 皮膚接觸試驗

pedicle 蒂

pedicle flap 有蒂皮瓣

pediculosis 虱病

pemphigus 天疱病

pemphigus vulgaris
尋常天疱瘡

phyllodes tumour 分葉狀腫瘤

pityriasis 糠疹

pityriasis alba 白糠疹

pityriasis rosea 玫瑰糠疹

pityriasis versicolor
  花斑糠疹 (汗斑癬)

porphyria 紫質症

position emission tomographic
  scan 正電子放射層照掃描

progesterone receptor
  孕激素受體

prolactin 催乳素

prurigo 癢疹

psoriasis 銀屑病 (牛皮癬)

puberty 發育期

purpura 紫癜

pustule 膿疱

pyogenicum, granuloma
  化膿性內芽腫

radiotherapy 放射治療

rash 疹

ring worm 癬

rosacea 玫瑰痤瘡，酒渣鼻

saline prosthesia 鹽水性義乳植
  入體

sarcoidosis 結節病

scabies 疥瘡，疥癩

scald 燙傷

scale 鱗屑

scar 疤

scarlet fever 腥紅熱

scleroderma 硬皮病

sebaceous cyst 皮脂囊腫 (粉瘤)

sebaceous gland 皮脂腺

sentine lymph mode biopsy
  前哨淋巴結組織檢查法

sexually transmitted disease
  性接觸傳染病

seborrhoeic keratosis
  皮脂性角化病

sentinel lymph node
  前哨淋巴結

shingles, herpes zoster
  帶狀疱疹

skeletal survey
  全身骨骼 X 光檢查

skin 皮 (膚)

skin biopsy 皮膚活組織檢驗

skin flap 皮瓣

skin flap, rotation 轉動皮瓣

skin graft 皮膚移植

skin graft, full thickness
  全層皮膚移植

skin graft, split thickness
  表層皮膚移植

skin test 皮膚(敏感)試驗

squamous cell carcinoma 鱗狀細胞癌

squamous epithelium 鱗狀上皮

staging of tumour 腫瘤分期鑑定

stereotactic biopsy 立體取組織檢查法

subcutaneous tissue 皮下組織

sweat gland 汗腺

syphilis 梅毒

syphilis, chancre 梅毒下疳(硬疳)

syphilis, gumma 梅毒瘤

syphilis, primary 初期梅毒

syphilis, secondary 二期梅毒

syphilis, late 後期梅毒

systemic lupus erythematosus (SLE) 紅斑性狼瘡 (擴散性紅斑狼瘡)

targeted therapy 標靶治療

telangiectasia 微絲血管擴張

tinea 癬

tinea cruris 股癬

tinea pedis 腳癬(香港腳)

tinea rubrum 紅核癬

tinea versicolor 花斑癬(汗斑癬)

transverse rectus abdominis myocutaneous (TRAM) flap 腹直肌皮瓣橫向移植術

tuberculosis (TB) 結核(病)

ulcer 潰瘍

ulcer, decubitus 褥瘡性潰瘍

ulcer, presacral 骶骨前潰瘍

ulcer, stasis (郁)鬱血性潰瘍

ulcer, varicose 靜脈曲張性潰瘍

ultrasound guided 超聲波引

ultraviolet light therapy 紫外光療法

urticaria 蕁麻疹(風疹塊)

vacuum assisted biopsy 真空輔助活組織檢驗

vasculitis 血管炎

verruca vulgaris 尋常疣

vitiligo 白斑(白蝕)

wart 疣

wheal 條痕

xanthelasma 黃斑瘤

xanthoma 黃瘤

zinc paste 鋅糊劑

6 **Circulatory System** 循環系統

abdominal aortic aneurysm
腹主動脈瘤

above knee amputation
膝關節上截肢術

acute cardia tamponade
急性心包填塞

acute heart failure 急性心功能
不全或急性心力衰竭

amputation 截肢術

aneurysm
動脈瘤 (動脈瘤形膨脹)

aneurysm, aortic 主動脈瘤

aneurysm, cerebral artery
大腦動脈瘤

aneurysm, dissecting
割裂性動脈瘤

aneurysm, false 假性動脈瘤

aneurysm, mycotic 動脈瘤，真
菌引起的

aneurysm, ruptured
動脈瘤破裂

aneurysm, thoracoabdominal
胸腹動脈瘤

aneurysm sinus of Valsalva
華沙華氏竇瘤

aneurysmectomy
動脈瘤切除術

angina pectoris 心絞痛

angiogram/arteriogram
動脈造影

angiogram, abdominal aorta
腹主動脈造影

angiogram, aortic arch
主動脈弓造影

angiogram, carotid
頸動脈造影

angiogram, cerebral
腦動脈造影

angiogram, femoral
股動脈造影

angiogram, translumbar
經腰椎動脈造影

angioplasty 血管整形術

angioscopy 血管內窺鏡

annuloplasty 瓣環成形術

anticoagulant 抗凝藥

anticoagulation 抗凝

antihypertensive drug
抗高血壓藥

aorta 主動脈

**aortic dissection (Dissecting
 aneurysm)** 主動脈

aortitis 主動脈炎

arrhythmia 心律不規律，
心律不正

arteriole 小動脈

arteriosclerosis 動脈硬化

arteriovenous fistula 動靜脈瘤

arteriovenous shunting
動靜脈分流術

arteriovenous malformation
動靜脈畸形

arteritis 動脈炎

artery 動脈

artery, brachial 臂動脈

**artery, brachiocephalic
 (innominate)** 頭臂動脈
（無名動脈）

artery, carotid, common
頸總動脈

artery, carotid, external
頸外動脈

artery, carotid, internal
頸內動脈

artery, cerebral 大腦動脈

artery, coeliac 腹腔動脈

artery, coronary 冠狀動脈

artery, digital 指（趾）動脈

artery, femoral, common
股總動脈

artery, femoral, profunda
股深動脈

artery, femoral, superficial
股淺動脈

artery, gastric 胃動脈

artery, hepatic 肝動脈

artery, iliac, common
髂總動脈

artery, iliac, external 髂外動脈

artery, iliac, internal 髂內動脈

artery, mesenteric, inferior
腸系膜下動脈

artery, mesenteric, superior
腸系膜上動脈

artery, popliteal 膕動脈

artery, pulmonary 肺動脈

artery, radial 橈動脈

artery, renal 腎動脈

artery, subclavian 鎖骨下動脈

artery, tibial 脛動脈

artery, ulnar 尺動脈

asystole 心跳停止

atherosclerosis 血管硬化症

atresia 閉鎖

atrial appendage 心房附件

atrial myxoma 心房粘液瘤

atrial septal defect
心房間隔缺損

atrium 心房

auscultation 聽診

B adrenergic receptor
blockade
B 腎上腺素受體阻斷藥

ballon angioplasty
球囊擴張

below knee amputation
膝關節下截肢術

blood flow 血流量

blood pressure 血壓

blood pressure, diastolic
心舒血壓

blood pressure, systolic
心縮血壓

blood vessel 血管

brachytherapy
近距離放射治療

bradycardia 心動過媛

bruit 雜音

Buerger's disease
(thromboangiitis obliterans)
閉塞形脈管炎

Budd-Chiari syndrome 布加綜
合症

bypass 分流術，搭橋分流

capillary 毛細血管

capillary hemangioma 毛細血
管瘤

cardiac arrest 心跳驟停

cardiac catheterization
心導管術

cardiac enzyme 心肌酶

cardiac massage 心臟按摩術

cardiac output 心血輸出量

cardiac tamponade 心包填塞

cardiectomy 心臟切除術

cardiogenic shock 心原性休克

cardiology/cardiologist
心臟科／心臟醫生

cardioplegic solution
心臟停跳液

cardiomegaly 心臟肥大

cardiomyopathy 心肌病

cardiopulmonary bypass
體外循環

cardioversion 心律正常化

carotid angioplasty
頸動脈失術

carotid stenosis 頸動狹窄症

carotid endarterectomy 頸動
脈內膜切除術

catheter 導管

cavenous hemangioma 海綿狀
血管瘤

central venous pressure
中心靜脈壓

cervical sympathectomy
頸交感神經切除術

**cerebral vascular accident
(CVA)** 腦血管意外 (中風)

chordae tendineae 腱索

chronic cardiac tamponade
慢性心包填塞

chronic heart failure
慢性心功能不全，
慢性心力衰竭

chronic venous insufficiency
慢性靜脈瓣膜功能不全

cine fluoroscopy
X 光透視 (電影)

cine-angiocardiography
心血管活動造影 (電影心血管
造影術)

circulation 循環

circulation, collateral
側支循環

circulation, portal 門脈循環

coarctation of aorta
主動脈縮窄

coil embolization

conduction 傳導

congenital 先天性

congestive heart failure
充血性心力衰竭

cor pulmonale
肺源性心臟病 (肺心病)

**coronary artery bypass
grafting** 冠狀動脈架橋術

cover stent 帶膜支架

CT angiogram CT 血管造影

cyanosis 發紫，發紺

deep venous system
深靜脈系統

deep vein reconstruction 深靜
脈重健術

deep vein thrombosis
深靜脈血栓形成

defibrillation 電除顫

dextrocardia 右位心

diastole 舒張期

digital subtraction angiography (DSA) 電腦數碼相減血管造數，數字減影血管造影

digitalis 洋地黃 （毛地黃，強心藥）

disseminated intravascular coagulopathy (DIC) 播散性血管內凝血機制障礙

diuretic 利尿劑

doppler studies 多卜勒檢查，超音波血流檢查

dyspnoea 呼吸困難

dyspnoea at rest 靜止時呼吸困難

dyspnoea on exertion 運動時呼吸困難

echocardiogram 超音波心臟掃描術

electrocardiogram (ECG) 心電圖

embolectomy 栓子切除術

embolus 栓子

embolus, air 氣栓子

embolus, clot 凝血栓子

embolus, fat 脂栓子

endarterectomy 動脈內壁膜切除術

endocarditis 心內膜炎

endocardium 心內膜

endoleak 內漏

endovastcular aortic stent graft 主動脈腔內支架治療

endovascular stent 血管內腔內支架

endovascular surgery 腔內血管外科技術

endovascular therapy 腔內血管治療

epicardium 心外膜

extra anatomic bypass 解剖外旁路移植術

extracorporeal circulation 體外循環

fibrillation 纖維性顫動

fibrillation, atrial 心房纖維性顫動

fibrillation, ventricular 心室纖維性顫動

first heart sound 第一心音

fistula 瘻管

fluoroscopy X 光透視

foramen ovale 卵圓窩

gangrene 壞疽，壞死

graft 移植，移植物

graft, artificial 人工移植

graft, vein 靜脈移植

guide wire 導絲

haemangioma 血管瘤

haemorrhae 出血

heart 心臟

heart block 心傳導阻滯

heart block, first degree
一度傳導阻滯

heart block, second degree
二度傳導阻滯

heart block, third degree
三度傳導阻滯

heart failure
心力衰竭、心功能不全

heart transplantation
心臟移植

heart valve replacement
心瓣替換

heart-lung transplantation
心肺聯合移植

hemangioma 血管瘤

heparin 肝素

homograft valve 同種瓣膜

hyperhidrosis 肝腺分泌過量

hypertension 高血壓

hypertension, pulmonary
肺動脈高壓症，肺循環高血壓

hypotension 低血壓

infarction 梗塞

intermittent claudication
間歇性跛行

interposition graft 交叉位移植

intra-aortic ballon pump
主動脈內氣球唧筒

ischaemia 缺血

IVC filter 下腔靜脈濾網

left ventricular failure
左心功能不全，左心衰

left ventricular rupture
左心室破裂

ligation 結紮

ligation and stripping
結紮與剝脫術

lipoprotein electrophoresis
脂蛋白電解分析

lumbar sympathectomy
腰交感神經切除術

lymphangiogram
淋巴管造影術

lymphoedema 淋巴水腫

MRA 磁力共振血管造影

mesenteric ishemia 腸系膜血管
供應不全

minimal extra corporeal
circulation (MECC)
術創體外循環技術

murmur 雜音

murmur, diastolic 舒張期雜聲

murmur, systolic 收縮期雜聲

myocardial infarction
　　心肌缺血敗壞

myocardial ischaemia
　　心肌缺血

myocardial protection
　　心肌保護

myocarditis 心肌炎

myocardium 心肌

normal sinus rhythm
　　正常竇性心律

open heart surgery
　　直視心臟手術

orthopnoea 端坐呼吸

oxygenation 氧合作用

pacemaker 心臟起搏器

pacemaker, epicardial
　　心外膜起搏器

pacemaker, transvenous
　　經靜脈起搏器

pallor 蒼白

palpitation 心悸

papillary muscle 乳頭狀肌

paroxysmal 陣發性

patch angioplasty 加膜血管
　　手術

patent ductus arteriosus
　　動脈導管不閉症

percutaneous 經皮穿刺

perforator vein 交通靜脈

pericardial effusion 心包積液

pericardiectomy 心包切除術

pericarditis 心包炎

pericardium 心包膜

pericardotomy 心包切開術

plethysmography
　　血流量圖測定體積

**popliteal entrapment
　syndrome** 膕血管陷迫綜合症

portal hypertension
　　門靜脈高壓症

pressure bandage 壓迫繃帶

pressure stocking 壓迫長襪

profundoplasty
　　肌深動脈形成術

prolapse 脫垂

pseudoaneurysm 假性動脈瘤

**pulmonary artery wedge
　pressure** 肺動脈嵌壓

pulmonary atresia 肺動脈閉鎖

pulmonary embolism 肺栓塞

pulse, irregular 不規則脈搏

pulse, peripheral 周圍脈搏

pulse, regular 規則脈搏

pulse rate 脈搏率

pulse volume 脈量

Raynaud's phenomenon
電諾氏現象

rebivascykar gtoertebsuib 腎血
管性高血壓

rest pain 靜止痛

rheumatic heart disease
風濕性心臟病

right ventricular failure
右心功能不全，右心衰

rT-PA 重組織綹溶酶原激活劑

rupture 破裂

sapheno-femoral flush ligation
大陰股平面血管結紮術

second heart sound 第二心音

serum cholesterol 血清膽固醇

serum triglyceride
血清三硝酸甘油酯

short of breath 呼吸短促

shunt 分流術

sinusoid 竇狀隙

sinus of Valsalva 華沙華氏竇

stent 支架

stent, coronary artery 冠狀動
脈支架

stent graft 帶膜支架

stent-graft endovascular 血管
內支架移植

stripping 剝脫

stroke 中風

subacute bacterial
endocarditis (SBE)
亞急性細菌性心內膜炎

subclavian steal sydnrome
鎖物下動脈潛行症狀

superficial venous system 淺靜
脈系統

sympathectomy
交感神經切斷術

systole 心收縮期

tachycardia 心跳過速

tetralogy of Fallot 心四聯畸形

thoracic outlet syndrome
胸腔出口綜合症

thoracoabdominal aortic
aneurysm 胸腹主動脈瘤

thoracoscopy 胸腔窺鏡

thrill 震顫

thrombectomy 血栓切除術

thrombolytic therapy
溶栓療法

thrombophlebitis
血栓性靜脈炎

thrombosis 淤塞

transient ischaemic attack
(TIA) 短暫性腦缺血

transposition of great vessels
大血管轉位

tricuspid atresia 三尖瓣閉鎖

truncus arteriosus
共同動脈幹畸形

ulcer 潰瘍

ulcer, arterial 動脈性潰瘍

ulcer, venous stasis
靜脈停滯性潰瘍

ulcer, venous varicose
靜脈曲張性潰瘍

urokinase 尿激酶

valve 心瓣

valve prolapse 瓣膜脫垂

valve, aortic 主動脈瓣

valve, atresia 心瓣閉鎖

valve, insufficiency
心瓣閉鎖不全

valve, mitral (bicuspid) 二尖瓣

valve, pulmonary 肺動脈瓣

valve, regurgitation
心瓣血回流

valve, stenosis 心瓣狹窄

valve, tricuspid 三尖瓣

valve replacement 瓣膜替換術

valvotomy 瓣膜切開術

varices 靜脈曲張

varices, oesophageal
食道靜脈曲張

varices, saphenous 隱靜脈曲張

vasculitis 血管炎

vasodilatation 血管舒張

vasodilating drug 血管舒張藥

vegetation 贅生物

vein 靜脈

vein, deep 深部靜脈

vein, femoral 股內靜脈

vein, hepatic 肝靜脈

vein, iliac, common 髂總靜脈

vein, iliac, external 髂外靜脈

vein, iliac, internal 髂內靜脈

vein, jugular, external
頸外靜脈

vein, jugular, internal
頸內靜脈

vein, perforating 穿靜脈

vein, portal 門靜脈

vein, pulmonary 肺靜脈

vein, saphenous, long 大隱靜脈

vein, saphenous, short
小隱靜脈

vein, subclavian 鎖骨下靜脈

vein, varicose 靜脈曲張

vena azygos 奇靜脈

vena cava, inferior 下腔靜脈

vena cava, superior 上腔靜脈

venae comitantes 並行靜脈

ventricle 心室

ventricular assist device
心室輔助裝置

ventricular dilatation
心室擴大

ventricular hypertrophy
心室肥大

ventricular septal defect
心室間隔缺損

venule 小靜脈

xenograft 異種移植

Respiratory System 呼吸系統

abscess 膿腫 (瘡)

acid-base balance 酸鹼平衡

adrenaline 腎上腺素

acute respiratory distress syndrome
急性呼吸窘迫綜合症

aerosol 氣霧藥

airway 呼吸道，空氣通道

allergy 變態反應 (過敏)

alveolus 肺泡

antibiotic 抗菌素 (抗生素)

arterial blood gas 動脈血氣壓

asbestosis 石棉肺

aspergillosis 麴菌病

asphyxia 窒息

aspiration 吸入

asthma 哮喘

asthma, extrinsic 外引性哮喘

asthma, intrinsic 內引性哮喘

asthmaticus, status
哮喘持續狀態

atelectasis 肺膨脹不全

atopic 無反應，離位

auscultation 聽診

bifurcation 分叉

biopsy 活組織檢驗 (活檢)

biopsy, lung
肺活組織檢驗 (肺活檢)

biopsy, pleura
胸膜活組織檢驗 (胸膜活檢)

bronchiectasis 支氣管擴張

bronchial challenge
支氣管功能測試

bronchiole 小支氣管

bronchiolitis 小支氣管炎

bronchitis 支氣管炎

bronchodilator 支氣管擴張藥

bronchogenic cyst 支氣管囊腫

bronchogram 支氣管造影

bronchopleural fistula
支氣管胸膜瘻管

bronchoscopy 支氣管鏡檢查

bronchospasm 支氣管痙攣

bronchus 支氣管

bullae 肺大疱

carbon monoxide poisoning
一氧化碳中毒

carcinoma, lung 肺癌

chest drain 胸膜引流

chest pain 胸痛

chronic bronchitis
慢性支氣管炎

**chronic obstructive
pulmonary disease (COPD)**
慢性氣管阻塞病

chyle 乳糜

chylothorax
胸膜積乳糜 (乳糜胸)

cilia 纖毛

clavicle 鎖骨

clubbing of fingers 杵狀指

collapse, lung 肺萎陷

compliance 順應性

**computerized axial
tomography (CAT)**
電腦軸切層造影

**continuous positive airway
pressure (CPAP)**
繼續性氣道正壓

cor pulmonale
肺源性心臟病 (肺性心病)

coronavirus 冠狀病毒

corticosteroid 腎上腺皮層素

costal cartilage 肋軟骨

costophrenic angle 脊肋角

cough 咳 (嗽)

crepitation 捻髮聲，輾軋聲

cyanosis 發紫，發紺

cytology 細胞學，細胞檢驗

cytology, exfoliative
脫落細胞檢驗

decortication 皮質剝脫術

desensitization 脫敏 (感)

diaphragm 橫隔膜

diaphragmatic hernia
橫膈膜疝

diaphragmatic irritation
橫膈膜刺激

dyspnoea 呼吸困難

embolus 栓子

embolus, air 氣栓子

embolus, clot 凝血栓子

embolus, fat 脂栓子

emphysema 肺氣腫

empyema thoracis
胸膜積膿 (膿胸)

endotracheal intubation
喉內插管

exercise testing 活動測試

exercise tolerance 運動耐力

expectorant 喀痰藥

expiration 呼氣

fibreoptic 光纖維

fibrosis 纖維化

filtration 過濾

flail chest 胸壁不穩

flu 流行性感冒

forced expiratory volume in 1
second (FEV1)
一秒鐘強力呼出量

forced vital capacity (FVC)
勁力肺活量

foreign body 異物

friction rub 胸膜磨擦聲

gas exchange 氣交替

granuloma 肉芽

haemoptysis 咳血

haemothorax 胸膜積血 (血胸)

hilum 肺門

hoarseness 聲嘶

hypercapnia 高血碳酸

hypersensitivity 過敏性

hyperventilation 呼吸過度

hypoxaemia 低血氧

hypoxia 缺氧

infiltrate 浸潤

influenza 流行性感冒

inhalation 吸入

inspiration 吸氣

intercostal 肋間

intercostal muscle 肋間肌

intercostal nerve 肋間神經

intercostal nerve block
肋間神經麻醉

intercostal retraction 肋間凹陷

kyphosis 脊柱後彎

laryngitis 喉炎

laryngoscopy 喉鏡檢查

larynx 喉

lobectomy 肺葉切除術

lung 肺

lung abscess 肺膿腫

lung scan
　　肺放射性素描 (肺素描)

mediastinitis 縱膈炎

mediastinoscopy 縱膈鏡檢查

mediastinum 縱膈

mesothelioma 間皮癌

metered dose inhalers
　　吸入劑量

mucolytic agent 黏液溶解藥

mycotic infection 霉菌感染

nebulizer 噴霧器

obstructive sleep apnoea
　　阻塞性睡眠窒息
opportunistic infection
　　投機性感染
oximetry 血液氧飽和度測試術

oxygen 氧氣

oxygen concentrator
　　氧濃度測試儀
oxygen saturation (SaO$_2$)
　　氧飽和

peak expiratory flow rate
　　呼氣最高流量
peak flow meter
　　呼吸最高流量測量儀
perfusion 灌注

pharyngitis 咽炎

phrenic nerve 膈 (膜) 神經

physiotherapy 物理治療

pleura 胸膜

pleura, parietal 壁層胸膜

pleura, visceral 臟層胸膜

pleural cavity 胸膜腔

pleural effusion 胸膜積液

pleuritic pain 胸膜痛

pleuritis 胸膜炎

pleurodesis 胸膜黏合

pneumococcus 肺炎球菌

postion emission tomography
　　正電子 (放射)
pneumocystis carinii
　　pneumonia
　　實質性血漿細胞肺炎
pneumonectomy 肺切除術

pneumonia (pneumonitis) 肺炎

pneumonia, atypical
非典型性肺炎

pneumonia, bacterial 細菌肺炎

pneumonia, broncho-
支氣管炎

pneumonia, lobar 肺葉炎

pneumonia, virus
過濾性菌肺炎

pneumoniae, Mycoplasma
支原體肺炎

pneumothorax
胸膜積氣 (氣胸)

pneumothorax, spontaneous
自發性氣胸

pneumothorax, tension
壓迫性氣胸

polycythaemia 血紅細胞增多

positive-end-expiratory
pressure (PEEP) 呼氣正壓端

postural drainage 體位引流法

pulmonary angiogram
肺脈造影

pulmonary artery 肺動脈

pulmonary embolus 肺脈栓子

pulmonary function test
肺功能檢查

pulmonary hypertension
肺脈高壓

pulmonary infarction
肺缺血敗壞

pulmonary rehabilitation
肺功純康復

pneumoconiosis
肺塵埃沉著病 (塵肺)

pulmonary oedema 肺水腫

pulmonary vein 肺靜脈

rales 羅聲

respiration 呼吸

respiratory failure 呼吸衰竭

rhinitis 鼻炎

rhonchi 干囉聲

rib 肋骨

rib fracture 肋骨折斷

sarcoidosis 肉樣瘤病

scapula 肩胛骨

scoliosis 脊椎側凸

segment 節

severe acute respiratory
syndrome (SARS)
急性嚴重呼吸綜合症

silicosis 矽肺病

skin test 皮層感應試驗

smear 抹片

spirometry 肺活量測定法

sputum 痰

sternum 胸骨

stethoscope 聽診器 (聽筒)

stridor 喘鳴

tachypnoea 氣促，呼吸急促

thoracic cavity 胸腔

thoracic vertebra 胸椎

thoracocentesis 胸腔穿刺術

thoracoscopy 胸腔窺鏡

thoracotomy 胸腔割開術

thorax 胸

thymus 胸腺

tidal volume 潮式量

tomography 切層造影

trachea 氣管

tracheitis 氣管炎

tracheostomy 氣管造口術

transfer factor 轉變因素

tuberculin test 結核菌質試驗

tuberculosis (TB) 結核 (病)

tuberculosis, miliary
粟粒性結核病

turbuhaler 渦輪噴射吸入器

upper respiratory tract infection (URI)
上呼吸道感染

ventilation 呼吸，換氣

ventilation and perfusion scans 通氣與灌注量掃描

ventilation, mechanical
人工換氣機

venturi mask 氣流式面窩

vital capacity 肺活量

wheeze 哮鳴

8 **Digestive System** 消化系統

α-fetoprotein 甲胎蛋白

24 hr pH monitoring 24 小時酸性強度

abdominal perineal resection of rectum 肛門直腸切除術

abdominal wall 腹壁

abdominal X-ray 腹部 X 光

abscess 膿腫

abscess, appendicular 闌尾膿腫

abscess, intrahepatic 肝臟內膿腫

abscess, ischiorectal 坐骨直腸膿腫

abscess, pancreatic 胰臟內膿腫

abscess, pelvic 盆腔膿腫

abscess, perianal 肛周膿腫

abscess, subphrenic 膈下膿腫

achalasia 張力失調、弛緩不能

adenocarcinoma 腺癌

adenoma 腺瘤

adenoma, villous 絨毛腺瘤

adhesion 粘連

aerophagia 吞氣症

alanine amino transferase ALT 丙氨酸氨基轉移酶

alcoholic liver disease 酒精毒性肝病

alcoholism 酒精中毒

alkaline phosphatase 碱性磷酸酶

ambulatory 24 hour pH monitoring test 動態24小時 pH監測

amoebiasis (amoebic dysentery) 阿米巴痢疾

ampulla of Vater 總膽管出口

amylase 澱粉酶

anal fissure 肛裂

anal sphincter 肛門括約肌

anal wart 肛門疣

anastomosis 接駁

anastomotic ulcer 接駁口潰瘍

angiodysplasia 血管營成異常

anorexia 厭食 (無胃口)

antacid 抗酸藥

antacid therapy 抗酸治療

anterior resection of rectum 直腸切除術

anticholinergic drug 抗膽素激導藥

antidiarrhoeal drug 抗瀉藥

antiemetic drug 止嘔吐藥

antiviral therapy 抗病毒治療

anus 肛門

appendicectomy 闌尾切除術

appendicitis 闌尾炎

artery 動脈

artery, coeliac 腹腔動脈

artery, gastric 胃動脈

artery, hepatic 肝動脈

artery, inferior mesenteric 下腸系膜動脈

artery, superior mesenteric 上腸系膜動脈

ascaris 蛔蟲

ascites 腹水

aspartate amino-transferase AST 天冬氨酸氨基轉移酶

aspiration 吸入，吸引

assimilation 同化

bacteria 細菌

banding, endoscopic 內視鏡綁紮法

barium enema 鋇灌腸造影

barium meal 鋇餐造影

barium swallow 鋇吞咽造影

Barrett's esophageal 巴雷特食管

belching 噯氣

bezoar 毛糞石

bile 膽液

bile duct 膽管

bilirubin 膽紅質

bilirubin, conjugated 結合後膽紅質

bilirubin, unconjugated 未結合膽紅質

biopsy 活(體)組織檢查

blind loop 盲腸環

bypass 支流術

bypass, double
食管雙重支流術

caecostomy 盲腸造口術

caecum 盲腸

calorie 卡

calorie, high 高卡,高熱量

calorie, low 低卡,低熱量

carbon-[13] Urea Breath test
碳[13]-尿素呼吸試驗

carcinoid tumour 類癌腫瘤

carcinoma 癌

carcinoma, colon 結腸癌

carcinoma, gastric 胃癌

carcinoma, liver 肝癌

carcinoma, oesophagus 食管癌

carcinoma, pancreas 胰癌

cardia 賁口

cardio-oesophageal junction
食管賁口接點

cathartic 瀉藥

cholangiogram 膽管造影

cholangiogram, intravenous
靜脈注射膽管造影

cholangiogram, percutaneous transhepatic
穿皮透肝膽管造影

cholangiogram, retrograde
逆行注射膽管造影

cholangitis 膽管炎

cholangitis, recurrent pyogenic 復發化膿性膽管炎

cholecystectomy 膽囊切除術

cholecystitis 膽囊炎

cholecystitis, acute 急性膽囊炎

cholecystitis, chronic
慢性膽囊炎

cholecystitis, gangrenous
壞疽性膽囊炎

cholecystogram, oral 膽囊造影

choledocholithiasis 膽管石病

choledochoscopy 膽管鏡

cholelithiasis 膽石病

cholestasis 膽汁鬱滯

chyle 乳糜

cirrhosis 肝硬化

cirrhosis, alcoholic
酒精性肝硬化

cirrhosis, biliary 膽汁性肝硬化

cirrhosis, post hepatic
肝炎後肝硬化

colectomy 結腸切除術

colectomy, right hemi-
右結腸部分切除術

colectomy, sigmoid
乙狀結腸切除術

colectomy, subtotal
次全結腸切除術

colectomy, total 全結腸切除術

colic 絞痛

colic, biliary 膽石絞痛

colitis 結腸炎

colitis, ischaemic 缺血結腸炎

colitis, ulcerative
潰瘍性結腸炎

colon 結腸

colon, ascending 升結腸

colon, descending 降結腸

colon, sigmoid 乙狀結腸

colon, transverse 橫結腸

colonoscopy 結腸鏡檢查

colostomy 結腸造口 (人造肛門)

common bile duct 膽總管

constipation 便秘

Crohn's disease
節段性回腸炎

cryotherapy 極凍冷療

cyst 水囊，囊腫

defaecation 排糞

deficiency 缺乏

deficiency, folic acid 葉酸缺乏

deficiency, iron 鐵質缺乏

deficiency, lactase 乳糖酶缺乏

deficiency, vitamin B12
維生素 B12 缺乏

diarrhoea, diarrhea 瀉

diet 飲食，減肥

diet, diabetic 糖尿病飲食

diet, fat free 無脂飲食

diet, high caloric 高熱量飲食

diet, high fibre 多纖維飲食

diet, high protein 高蛋白飲食

diet, high residue 高渣飲食

diet, light 易消化飲食

diet, liquid 流質飲食

diet, low sodium 低鈉飲食

diet, soft 軟飲食

diet, vegetarian 植物性飲食

digestion 消化

dissolution 溶解

dissolution of gall stone
膽石溶解

diuretic 利尿劑

diverticulitis 憩室炎

diverticulosis 憩室病

diverticulum 憩室

diverticulum, colon 結腸憩室

diverticulum, Zenker
  掇食管內壓性憩室

duct 管，導管

duct, common bile 總膽管

duct, cystic 膽囊管

duct, hepatic 肝管

duct, pancreatic 胰管

dumping syndrome
  傾倒綜合微狀

duodenal ulcer 十二指腸潰瘍

duodenitis 十二指腸炎

duodenum 十二指腸

dyspepsia 消化不良

dysphagia 吞咽困難

dysplasia
  發育不良，不典型增生

**endoscopic retrograde
  cholangiopancreatography
  (ERCP)** 內窺鏡肝胰管造影

endoscopy 內視鏡

enterescopy 腸鏡

enteritis 腸炎

**enteritis, regional (Crohn's
  disease)** 間區性腸炎

enzyme 酶（酵素）

epigastrium 上腹

eructation 噯氣

esophagitis 食管炎

esophagogram 食管X線照相術

**exploration of common bile
  duct** 總膽管探查

familial polyposis coli
  家族性腺瘤，家族性結腸
  息肉病

fatty liver 脂肪肝

fissure 裂

fistula 瘻，瘻管

fistula, broncho-oesophageal
  支氣管食管瘻

fistula, tracheo-oesophageal
  氣管食管瘻

fistula-in-ano 肛門瘻

flapping tremor 手撥震顫

flatulence 腸胃氣積

flatus 腸胃氣，屁

fundus 底

gall bladder 膽囊

gangrene 壞疽

gastrectomy 胃切除術

gastrectomy, partial
  胃部分切除術

gastrectomy, subtotal
  胃大部分切除術

gastrectomy, total 全胃切除術

gastric acid analysis 胃酸分析

gastric antrum 胃竇

gastric body 胃身

gastric cardia 胃賁口

gastric emptying 胃排空

gastric fundus 胃底

gastric greater curve 胃大彎

gastric lesser curve 胃小彎

gastric pylorus 胃幽門

gastric ulcer 胃潰瘍

gastrin 胃酸激素

gastrin meal test
　胃酸激素餐檢驗

gastritis 胃炎

gastroenteritis 胃腸炎

gastroptosis 胃下垂

gastroscopy 胃鏡檢查

gastrostomy 胃造口術

gastro-esophageal reflux
　disease (GERD)
　胃-食管反流病

H₂ blocker 組織胺第二位阻體

haematemesis 嘔血

haemorrhoid 痔

haemorrhoid, prolapse 痔脱垂

haemorrhoidectomy 痔切除術

heart burn 火燒心、心口灼
　熱，胸口灼熱

Helicobacter pylori 幽門螺旋菌

hepatectomy 肝切除術

hepatic encephalopathy
　肝腦病

hepatic failure 肝功能衰竭

hepatic flexure 結腸右曲

hepatitis 肝炎

hepatitis antibody 肝炎抗體

hepatitis antigen 肝炎抗原

hepatitis A 甲類肝炎

hepatitis B 乙類肝炎

hepatitis B antigen
　乙類肝炎抗原

hepatitis C 丙類肝炎

hepatitis D 丁類肝炎

hepatitis E 戊類肝炎

hepatitis G 季類肝炎

hepatitis, drug-induced
　藥物引起肝炎

hepatitis, non A, non B
　非甲非乙類肝炎

hepatitis antibody 肝炎抗體

hepatitis antigen 肝炎抗原

hepatitis vaccine 肝炎疫苗

hepatomegaly 肝腫大

herbal medicine 中藥

hernia 疝

hernia, femoral 股疝

hernia, hiatus 膈裂孔疝

hernia, inguinal 腹股溝疝

hernia, umbilical 臍疝

ileostomy 迴腸造口術

ileum 迴腸

ileus 腸梗阻

ileus, mechanical
　機械性腸梗阻

ileus, paralytic 麻痺性腸梗阻

iliac fossa 骼窩

indigestion 消化不良

infestation 侵染

insulin stimulation test
　胰島素刺激檢驗

interferon 干擾素

intestinal obstruction 腸梗阻

intestinal tuberculosis 腸結核

intussusception 腸套疊 (套腸)

irritable bowel syndrome
　腸功能應激性綜合症

jaundice (icterus) 黃疸

jaundice, extrahepatic
　肝外黃疸

jaundice, haemolytic
　溶血性黃疸

jaundice, hepatic 肝性黃疸

jaundice, obstructive
　梗阻性黃疸

jaundice, pre-hepatic 肝前黃疸

jejunum 空腸

lactase deficiency 乳糖酶缺乏

lactulose 通便糖

laparoscopy 腹腔鏡檢查

laparotomy 剖腹術

lactulose 通便糖

laxative 輕瀉藥

leiomyoma 平滑肌瘤

leiomyosarcoma 平滑肌肉瘤

lipase 脂酶

liver 肝

liver transplant 肝移植

lysis of adhesion 黏連鬆解術

malabsorption 吸收不良

Mallory-Weiss syndrome
　賁口黏膜破裂綜合症

megacolon 巨結腸

melaena 黑糞症

melanosis coli 結腸黑變病

mesenteric thrombosis
腸系膜血栓形成

mesentery 腸系膜

metastasis 癌轉移

milk intolerance
乳類食物不耐受

mucosa 粘膜

mucus 粘液

myotomy 肌切開術

nasogastric suction 胃喉抽吸

nasogastric tube 胃管

nausea 噁心 (作悶)

non-steroidal anti-inflammatory drug (NSAID)
非類固醇消炎止痛藥

nutrition 營養

nutrition, intravenous
靜脈營養

nutrition, total parenteral (TPN) 全靜脈營養

obstruction 梗塞

occult blood 潛血

oesophagectomy, esophagectomy 食管切除術

oesophagitis, esophagitis
食管炎

oesophagitis, esophagitis, reflux 回流食管炎

oesophagostomy, esophagostomy 食管造口術

oesophagus, esophagus 食管

omentum 網膜

pancreas 胰

pancreatectomy 胰切除術

pancreatic cyst 胰囊腫

pancreatic duct 胰管

pancreatic function test
胰功能檢驗

pancreatic pseudocyst
胰偽囊腫

pancreatitis 胰炎

pepsin 胃蛋白酶

peptic ulceration 消化性潰瘍

per rectum 探肛，直腸檢查

percutaneous transhepatic biliary drainage (PTBD)
穿皮透肝膽液引流

percutaneous transhepatic cholangiogram (PTC)
穿皮透肝膽管造影

perianal abscess 肛周膿腫

peristalsis 蠕動

peritoneal lavage 腹腔灌洗

peritoneoscopy 腹腔鏡檢查

peritonitis 腹膜炎

Peutz-Jeghers syndrome (multiple polyposis) 空腸息肉綜合症

plication 摺疊術

polyp 息肉

portacaval shunt 門腔靜脈分流術

portal hypertension 門靜脈高壓

portal hypertensive gastropathy 門脈高壓性胃病變

portal pyaemia 化膿性門靜脈炎

portal vein 門靜脈

proctitis 直腸炎

prolapse rectum 直腸脫垂

pruritus ani 肛癢

pseudocyst 假囊腫

purgative 導瀉藥

pyloric stenosis 幽門狹窄

pyloroplasty 幽門整形術

pylorus 幽門

rapid urease test 快速尿素酶檢查

rectal examination 探肛，直腸檢查

rectal prolapse 直腸脫垂

rectocele 直腸突出

rectum 直腸

regurgitation 反肚

Ryle's tube (nasogastric tube) 胃管

scleroderma 硬皮病

sclerotherapy 硬化療法

serum amylase 血清澱粉酶

shunt 分流

shunt, mesocaval 腸系膜腔靜脈分流術

shunt, portacaval 門腔靜脈分流術

shunt, splenorenal 脾腎靜脈分流術

sigmoidoscopy 乙狀結腸鏡

sphincter 括約肌

sphincteroplasty 括約肌成形術

sphincterotomy 括約肌切開術

splash, succussion 擊水聲

splenic flexure 結腸左曲

splenomegaly 脾腫大

splenorenal shunt 脾腎靜脈分流術

staple gun 釘合機

stapler 釘合機

steatorrhoea 脂肪下痢

stomach 胃

stomatitis 口炎

stool 糞

stool, losse 稀糞

stool, mucous 粘液性糞

stool, pea soup 豆漿樣糞

stool, tarry 煤膠樣糞

stool, watery 水樣糞

strangulation 絞窄

stricture 狹窄

swallow 吞咽

telangiectasia 毛細血管擴張

tenderness 觸痛

tenderness, rebound 反跳觸痛

tenesmus 沉脹 (裏急後重)

total parenteral nutrition
全靜脈營養

transarterial (oily) chemoembolization (TACE or TOCE)
經動脈 (油性) 化學栓塞術

transjugular intrahepatic portosystemic stent-shunt (TIPS)
經頸靜脈肝內門脈合流術

trypsin 胰蛋白酶鈉

typhoid fever 傷寒

ulcer 潰瘍

ulcer, duodenal 十二指腸潰瘍

ulcer, gastric 胃潰瘍

ulcer, peptic 消化性潰瘍

ultrasonogram 超音波掃描

upper endoscopy 腸胃鏡檢查

urea breath test 尿素呼吸測試

vaccine 疫苗

vagal stimulus 迷走神經刺激

vagotomy 迷走神經切斷術

vagotomy, proximal gastric
近胃迷走神經切斷術

vagotomy, selective
選擇性迷走神經切斷術

vagotomy, truncal
迷走神經幹切斷術

vagus 迷走神經

valve 活門，瓣

varices 靜脈曲張

vein 靜脈

vein, gastric 胃靜脈

vein, hepatic 肝靜脈

vein, inferior mesenteric
下腸系膜靜脈

vein, portal 門靜脈

vein, superior mesenteric
上腸系膜靜脈

virus, viral 過濾性病菌 (病毒)

volvulus 腸扭轉

vomit 嘔吐

vomiting, bilious 膽性嘔吐

vomiting, faeculent 糞性嘔吐

vomiting, projectile
　射出性嘔吐

Whipple's disease 惠普爾病
　(腸原性脂肪代謝障礙)

Whipple's operation
　惠普爾手術 (根治性胰頭十二
　指腸切除術)

Whipple's test 惠普爾試驗
　(檢測肝功能)

Wilson's disease 威爾遜氏病
　(先天性銅代謝障礙病)

xylose absorption test
　木糖吸收檢驗

9 Urinary/Male Genital System
泌尿與男性生殖系統

abscess 膿腫 (瘡)

abscess, perinephric
  腎周 (圍) 膿腫

abscess, psoas 腰肌膿腫

agenesis
  繁殖力缺乏 (生育不全)

anuria 閉尿

ascending urethrogram 逆流尿
  道造影

balanitis 陰莖頭炎 (龜頭炎)

balanoposthitis 陰莖頭炎 (龜頭
  炎)

biopsy 活組織檢驗

bladder 膀胱

bladder, neurogenic
  神經原性膀胱

bladder, neurological
  dysfunction
  神經原性膀胱功能失調

bladder capacity 膀胱容量

bladder exstrophy 膀胱外翻

bladder neck 膀胱頸

bladder neck suspension 膀胱
  頸懸吊術

bougie 探條

bouginage 擴張通條

bulbourethral gland
  (Cowper's gland) 尿道球腺

calcium oxalate 草酸鈣

calculus 石，結石

calculus, bladder 膀胱石

calculus, renal 腎石

calculus, staghorn
　腎盂石 (鹿角樣腎盂石)

calyx 腎盞

carcinoma 癌

carcinoma, embryonal
　胚胎 (組織) 癌

carcinoma, epidermoid
　表皮樣癌

carcinoma, renal cell 腎細胞癌

carcinoma, transitional cell
　過渡性細胞癌

catheter, Foley 留置導尿管

catheter, urine 導尿管

chordee 陰莖前曲

chyluria 乳糜尿

circumcision 包皮切除術

claculus, ureteric 輸尿管石

clamydia 依原體

colocystoplasty
　結腸膀胱造形術

colony count 細菌鱗數

computed tomography
　urogram 電腦掃描尿道造影

condom 避孕套

conduit, gastric 胃造管道

conduit, ileal 腸造管道

continence 節禁

contusion 撞傷

copora cavernosum
　陰莖海綿體

corona 陰莖頭冠

creatinine, serum 血肌酸

creatinine clearance, serum
　血肌酸　消除率

cremasteric reflex 提睪反射

cryptorchidism 隱睪病

culture and sensitivity test
　細菌培殖與感應檢驗

cyst 囊腫，水囊

cyst, renal 腎囊腫

cystectomy 膀胱切除術

cystectomy, partial
　部分膀胱切除術

cystectomy, total
　全部膀胱切除術

cystitis 膀胱炎

cystitis, haemorrhagic
　出血性膀胱炎

cystitis, interstial
　間質性膀胱炎

cystitis, irradiation
　放射性膀胱炎

cystometrogram
　膀胱內壓描記圖

cystometry 膀胱內壓測量

cystoplasty 膀胱整形術

cystoplasty, augmentation
　膀胱增大整形術

cystoplasty, colo
結腸膀胱整形術

cystoplasty, gastro
胃膀胱整形術

cystoscopy 膀胱鏡檢查

cystostomy 膀胱造口術

cystostomy, suprapubic
骨弓上膀胱造口術

cysto-urethroscopy
(panendoscopy)
尿道膀胱鏡檢查

descending urethrogram
順流尿道造影

detrusor 逼尿肌

dialysis 透析 (洗腎)

dialysis, haemo 血液透析

dialysis, peritoneal 腹膜透析

diuresis 利尿 (去水)

diuretic 利尿藥

diversion 分流手術

diverticulum 支囊 (憩室)

duplex kidney 二元腎

dysuria 排尿困難

ejaculation 射精

ejaculation, premature
射精過早 (早泄)

ejaculation, retrograde
逆行射精

ejaculatory duct 射精管

electromyogram (EMG)
肌電圖

enuresis, nocturnal 夜遺尿

epididymis 附睪

epididymitis 附睪炎

epididymo-orchitis 睪丸附睪炎

epispadias 尿道上裂

erectile dysfunction
勃起功能障礙

erection 勃起 (竪起)

exenteration 腔臟切除術

exenteration, anterior pelvic
前盆腔臟切除術

exenteration, posterior pelvic
後盆腔臟切除術

exenteration, total pelvic
全盆腔臟切除術

flank tenderness
腰窩痛 (脇腹痛)

frequency 尿頻

gastric conduit 胃造膀胱術

gastrocystoplasty
胃膀胱整形術

glans penis 陰莖頭 (龜頭)

glomerulonephritis
腎小球性腎炎

glomerulonephritis, acute
急性腎小球性腎炎

glomerulonephritis, chronic
慢性腎小球性腎炎

glomerulonephritis, lupus
狼瘡腎小球性腎炎

glomerulonephritis, post-streptococcal
鏈球菌後遺腎小球性腎炎

glomerulus 腎血管球 (腎小球)

gonorrhoea, gonorrhea 淋病

granuloma inguinale
腹股溝肉芽腫

groin 腹股溝

gubernaculum 引帶

haematocele 鞘膜積血

haematuria 血尿

haemospermia 射精帶血

hernia 疝 (小腸氣)

hernia, direct 直疝

hernia, femoral 股疝

hernia, indirect 斜疝

hernia, inguinal 腹股溝疝

hernia, irreducible 不還納形疝

hernia, reducible 還納形疝

hernia, strangulated 絞扼形疝

herniorrhaphy 疝修補術

herpes 皰疹

hesitancy 小便躊躇 (不順)

hormone 激素 (內分泌)

hormone, follicular stimulating (FSH) 卵胞激素

hormone, luteinizing (LH)
黃體激素

horse-shoe kidney 馬蹄鐵形腎

hydrocele 鞘膜積水 (水囊)

hydronephrosis 腎盂積水

hydroureter 輸尿管積水

hypertrophy 增大

hypospadias 尿道下裂

ileal conduit 迴腸造膀胱

impotence 陽萎 (性無能)

incontinence 失禁

incontinence, stress 壓力性尿失禁

incontinence, urine 尿失禁

infertility 不育

infertility, primary 原發性不育

infertility, secondary
繼發性不育

inguinal canal 腹股溝管

intermittent catheterization 間歇導尿

intersex 雌雄間性

intravenous urogram
排泄性尿道造影 (靜脈注射泌
尿系統造影)

kidney 腎

litholapaxy 石碾碎清除術

lithotomy 石清除術

lithotripsy 碎石術

lithotripsy, electrohydraulic
電水壓碎石術

lithotripsy, extracorporeal
shock wave 體外振波碎石術

lithotripsy, ultrasonic
超音波碎石術

loin 腰

lymphangiogram 淋巴造影

lymphogranuloma inguinale
腹股溝淋巴肉芽腫

masturbation 手淫 (自瀆)

meatus 尿道口

nephrectomy 腎切除術

nephritis 腎炎

nephroblastoma 腎胚胎癌

nephrocalcinosis 腎鈣質沉著症

nephrology/nephrologist
腎病學/腎病學醫生

nephron 腎單位

nephrosis 腎變病

nephrostomy 腎造口術

nephrostomy drain
腎做口引流

nephrotic syndrome
腎變病綜合症

nephrotomogram 腎切層造影

nitrite 亞硝酸鹽

nocturia 夜尿

oedema, edema 水腫

oligospermia 精數減少

oliguria 少尿

orchidopexy 睪丸固定術

orchitis 睪丸炎

orchitis, mumps 腮腺性睪丸炎

orchitis, tuberculosis
結核性睪丸炎

paraphimosis 箝頓包莖

pelvo ureteric junction
腎盂輸尿管道接點

penis 陰莖 (陽具)

percutaneous
nephrolithotoripsy
穿皮透腎碎石術

perineum 會陰

Peyronie's disease 陰莖硬結

phimosis 包莖

phosphatase 磷酸脂酶

phosphatase, acid
  酸性磷酸脂酶

phosphatase, alkaline
  鹼性磷酸脂酶

polycystic 多囊

polyuria 多尿

posterior urethral valve 後尿
  道瓣膜

prepuce 包皮

prostate 前列腺 (攝護腺)

prostatectomy 前列腺切除術

prostatectomy, perineal
  經會陰前列腺切除術

prostatectomy, radical
  根治性前列腺切除術

prostatectomy, suprapubic
  恥骨上前列腺切除術

prostatectomy, transurethral
  經尿道前列腺切除術

prostatic biopsy
  前列腺活組織檢驗

prostatic hypertrophy, benign
  良性前列腺脹大

prostatic specific antigen
  前列腺專有抗原

prostatitis 前列腺炎

proteinuria 蛋白尿

pubic hair 陰毛

pyelolithotomy 腎盂石清除術

pyelonephritis 腎盂炎

pyelonephritis, tuberculosis
  腎結核炎

pyeloplasty 腎盂整形術

pyonephrosis 膿性腎炎

pyuria 膿尿

quantitative culture 定量細菌
  培養

rectal examination 肛診

reflux 回流，反流

rejection 排斥

residual urine 殘尿

renal arteriogram 腎血管造影

renal failure 腎功能衰竭

renal function test (RFT)
  腎功能檢驗

renal pelvis 腎盂

renal scan 放射性腎掃描

renal transplant 腎臟移植

retrograde catheterization
  逆行導管插入術

retrograde pyelogram
  逆行腎盂造影

retroperitoneal fibrosis
後腹膜纖維化症

scrotum 陰囊

sear, fibrosis 結巴

semen (seminal fluid) 精液

seminal vesicle 精囊

seminoma 精原細胞癌

sperm 精子

spermatic cord 精索

spermatocele 精子囊腫

spermatogenesis 精子形成

sphincter 括約肌

stenosis 狹窄

stent 固定模管

stricture 管道狹隘

syphilis 梅毒

syphilitic chancre 梅毒初瘡

syphilitic gumma 梅毒瘤

teratoma 畸胎瘤

testis 睪丸

testis, ectopic 異位睪丸

testis, retractile 返縮性睪丸

testis, undescended
高隱睪丸 (雄激素)

testosterone 睪丸素〔雄激素〕

tomogram 切層造影

torsion 精索扭轉

trabecula 小樑，柱狀

trabeculation 小樑形成

transitional cell 過渡細胞

transitional epithelium
過渡性上皮

tunica vaginalis 鞘膜

ultrafiltration 超濾法

ultrasound scan 超音波素描

uraemia 尿毒症

urea 尿素

ureter 輸尿管

ureterocele 輸尿管疝

ureterolithiasis 輸尿管結石

ureterolithotomy
輸尿管石切除術

ureteroscope 輸尿管鏡

urethra 尿道

urethral gland 尿道腺

urethritis 尿道炎

urtehritis, non-gonococcal
非淋病尿道炎

urethroplasty 尿道整形術

urethroscope 尿道鏡

urethrotomy 尿道割開術

uric acid 尿酸

urine culture 尿液細菌培養

urinalysis 尿分析

urinary obstruction 尿道梗阻

urinary retention 尿留滯

urination 排尿 (小便)

urine 尿

urine antiseptic 尿抗菌劑

urine specimen, catheter
    導管收集尿樣本

urine specimen, midstream
    尿中流樣本

urodynamics 尿流動力學

uroflowmetry 尿流率測定

urology/urologist
    泌尿外科/泌尿外科醫生

urostomy 尿造口

varicocele 精索靜脈曲張

vas deferens 輸精管

vasectomy 輸精管切紮術

vasogram 輸精管造影

vasovasostomy 輸精管接駁術

venereal disease 性病

verumontanum 精阜

vesico-ureteric junction
    膀胱輸尿管接點

vesico-ureteric reflux
    膀胱輸尿管反流

voiding cystogram
    膀胱排尿造影

10 Female Genital System/ Obstetrics
女性生殖系統與產科

abstinence 節制

adenoma 腺瘤

adnexa uteri 子宮附件

amenorrhoea 閉經

amniocentesis

amniography 胎膜造影

amniotic fluid 胎膜水 (羊水)

amniotic fluid embolism
　胎水栓塞

amniotic membrane 胎膜

amniotic sac 胎膜囊

antenatal care 產前護理

antepartum haemorrhage
　產前出血

anus 肛門

Apgar score 初生嬰兒健康評估

artificial insemination
　人工授精

atony 張力缺乏 (無收縮)

atony, uterine 子宮收縮無力

Bartholin's gland 前庭腺

bartholinitis 前庭腺炎

birth trauma 出生創傷

Braxton Hicks' contractions
　妊娠子宮收縮

caesarean section 剖腹產

caput 頭

carcinoma 癌

carcinoma, adeno 腺癌

carcinoma, chorio 絨膜癌

carcinoma, cyst adeno 囊腺癌

carcinoma, embryonal
胚胎(組織)癌

carcinoma, squamous cell
鱗狀細胞癌

carcinoma, transitional cell
過渡性細胞癌

cephalopelvic disproportion
頭盆不稱

cervical biopsy
子宮頸活組織檢驗

cervical os 子宮口

cervix uteri 子宮頸

chemotherapy 藥物療法

chorionic villus biopsy

chromosome 染色體

climacteric 更年期

clinical staging 臨床分期

clitoris 陰蒂

clomiphene citrate
卵巢刺激素(多產丸)

coitus 性交

coitus interruptus
間斷式性交(體外射精)

colostomy 結腸造口(人造肛門)

colporrhaphy 陰道重整術

colposcopy 陰道鏡檢查

condom 避孕套

condyloma acuminatum
尖形濕疣

contraception 避孕

contraception, safety period
安全期避孕

contraceptive 避孕藥

contraction 收縮

convulsion 搐溺，痙攣，驚厥

corpus luteum 黃體

corpus uteri 子宮體

cortex 皮質

culdocentesis
子宮後陷凹抽樣本

culdoscopy 陷凹鏡檢查

cystocele 膀胱疝

cystometrogram
膀胱壓力描記圖

delivery 接生

delivery, forceps 產鉗接生

delivery, spontaneous 順產

delivery, vacuum extraction
真空吸引助產

descensus 胎下降

dilatation 宮口擴張

dilatation and curettage 刮宮

discharge 排泌(分泌)

discharge, bloody 染血排泌

discharge, purulent 含膿排泌

discharge, serous 漿液性排泌

Down syndorome 唐氏綜合症

dysmenorrhoea, essential
  自發性經痛

dysmenorrhoea, functional
  機能性經痛

dysmenorrhoea, secondary
  繼發性經痛

dyspareunia 性交疼痛

dysplasia 增殖異常

dystocia 難產

eclampsia 子癇

ectopic pregnancy 宮外孕

embryo transfer 胎兒較位

endometrial biopsy
  子宮內膜活組織檢驗

endometrial polyp
  子宮內膜息肉

endometriosis 子宮內膜異位

endometritis 子宮內膜炎

endometrium 子宮內膜

endopelvic fascia 骨盤內筋膜

enterocoele, enterocele
  陰道腸疝

episiotomy 會陰割開術

erythroblastosis fetalis
  胎紅血球病

estrogen 雌激素

exenteration 腔臟切除術

exenteration, anterior
  前盆腔臟切除術

exenteration, posterior
  後盆腔臟切除術

exenteration, total
  全盆腔臟切除術

**expected date of confinement
(EDC)** 預產期

fallopian tube 輸卵管

fibroma 纖維瘤

fimbria 輸卵管邊毛

fistula 瘻管

follicle stimulating hormone
  濾泡激素

**gonadotrophin-releasing
  hormone** 促性腺激素

hormone 激素

**human menopausal
  gonadotrophin (hMG)**
  人體收經期促性激素

hydramnios 胎水過多

hydrosalpinx 輸卵管積水

hymen 處女膜

hyperplasia 增殖

hypertension 高血壓

hypothalamus 下丘腦

hysterectomy 子宮切除術

hysterectomy, abdominal
剖腹子宮切除術

hysterectomy, laparoscopic assisted
腹腔鏡協助子宮切除術

hysterectomy, radical
徹底子宮切除術

hysterectomy, vaginal
經陰道子宮切除術

hysterosalpingography
子宮輸卵管造影

hysterotomy 子宮割開術

ileal conduit 迴腸人工膀胱

impaired glucose tolerance

in vitro **fertilization (IVF)**
體外受孕 (試管嬰兒)

incontinence 失禁

incontinence, faecal 大便失禁

incontinence, stress
壓迫下失禁

incontinence, stress urine
壓迫下尿失禁

incontinence, urine 尿失禁

infertility 不育

infertility, primary 原發性不育

infertility, secondary
繼發性不育

intertrigo 擦疹

intra-uterine contraceptive device (IUCD)
宮內節育器 (子宮環)

intracytoplasmic sperm injection 細胞漿內注精子

intrauterine insemination (IUI) 子宮內受精

karyotype 核內型

labia majora 大陰唇

labia minora 小陰唇

labour, labor 分娩，生產

labour, induction 引產

labour, premature 早產

laceration 撕裂

lactation 產乳

laparoscopy 腹腔鏡檢查

laparotomy 剖腹

last menstrual period
最後一次經期

leiomyoma (fibroid)
子宮纖維性平滑肌瘤
(纖維肌瘤)

levator sling 提肌，懸帶

libido 性慾

lie 胎位

lie, longitudinal 直置胎位

lie, transverse 橫置胎位

luteinizing hormone (LH)
黃體激素

lymphogranuloma venereum
(LGV) 花柳性淋巴肉芽腫

malformation 畸形

malformation, congenital
先天性畸形

masturbation 手淫 (自瀆)

maternal mortality rate
孕婦死亡率

membranes, premature
repture of 胎膜過早穿破

menarche 初經

menopausal, post- 閉經後

menopausal, pre- 閉經前

menopause 閉經 (收經)

menorrhagia 月經過多

menstrual cycle 經期

menstrual history 月經情況

menstruation 月經，行經

menstruation, menstrual cycle
經期

metrorrhagia 子宮過量出血

miscaniage 流產 (小產，墮胎)

miscaniage, habitual
習慣性流產

miscaniage, incomplete
不完全流產

miscaniage, induced
引發流產 (人工流產)

miscaniage, spontaneous
自發流產

miscaniage, threatened
先兆流產

miscarriage 流產

mortality rate 死亡率

mortality rate, infant
嬰兒死亡率 (一歲以下)

mortality rate, maternal
孕婦死亡率

mortality rate, neonatal
新生期嬰兒死亡率 (一月以下)

mortality rate, perinatal
產期嬰兒死亡率 (一週以下)

mucosa 黏膜

mucus 黏液

multiparity 多產

myoma 肌瘤

neonatal mortality rate
新生期嬰兒死亡率

obstruction 阻塞

oligohydramnios 胎水過少

oocyte retrieval 卵巢分裂遲緩

oophorectomy 卵巢切除術

oral contraceptive 口服避孕藥

os 子宮口

ovarian cyst 卵巢水瘤

ovary 卵巢

ovulation 排卵

oxytocic agent 催產藥

Pap smear
　子宮頸細胞抹片檢驗

parametria 子宮旁組織

parity 經產數目

patent 暢通

pelvic examination 婦科檢查

pelvic inflammatory disease
　盆腔炎

perinatal mortality rate
　產期嬰兒死亡率

perineum 會陰

pessary 子宮托

pituitary 腦下垂體

placenta 胎盤

placenta, abruption
　胎盤早期脱離

placenta, accreta 植入性胎盤

placenta, retention of
　胎盤滯留

placenta praevia 胎盤前置

polyp 息肉

post partum 產後

post partum haemorrhage
　產後流血

post partum ligation of tubes
　產後輸卵管結紮術

pouch of Douglas 子宮後陷凹

pre-eclampsia 先兆子癇

pregnancy 妊娠

premenstrual tension
　經前精神緊張

prenatal diagnosis 產前診斷

presentation 先露

presentation, abnormal
　異常先露

presentation, breech 臀先露

presentation, brow 額先露

presentation, cephalic 頭先露

presentation, face 面先露

presentation, foot 腳先露

presentation, hand 手先露

presentation, normal 正常先露

presentation, occiput 枕先露

presentation, occiput posterior
　枕後先露

presentation, occiput
　posterior, left 左枕後先露

presentation, shoulder 肩先露

primigravida 初孕

progesterone 黃體酮

promiscuous 濫交

prostaglandin 前列腺素

proteinuria 蛋白尿

pruritus 痕癢

pruritus vulva 女陰癢

puberty 發育期

pubic pediculosis 恥虱病

pyelonephritis 腎盂炎

pyosalpinx 輸卵管積膿

radiotherapy 放射治療

rectal examination 肛門檢查

rectocele 陰道直腸疝

renal function test 腎功能檢驗

rubella 風疹 (德國麻疹)

salpingitis 輸卵管炎

salpingitis, acute 急性輸卵管炎

salpingitis, chronic
  慢性輸卵管炎

salpingo-oophorectomy
  卵巢輸卵管切除術

sarcoma 肉癌

scabies 疥瘡

semen analysis 精虫分類

sexual behaviour 性行為

subfertility 受孕率低

sterilization 絕育

syphilis 梅毒

testosterone 睪丸素

thalassaemia
  地中海形血紅素貧血

tubal ligation 輸卵管結紮

tubal ligation, laparoscopic
  腹鏡輸卵管結紮

tubal ligation, post partum
  產後輸卵管結紮

tubo-ovarian abscess
  卵巢與輸卵管膿腫

twin 雙胞胎

**ultrasound scan,
  ultrasonography**
  超聲波掃描

umbilical cord 臍帶

umbilical cord, prolapse of
  臍帶脫垂

umbilicus 肚臍

urethra 尿道

urethrocele 陰道尿道疝

uterine prolapse 子宮脫垂

uterus 子宮

uterus, anteflexed 子宮前屈

uterus, anteverted 子宮前傾

uterus, retroflexed 子宮後屈

uterus, retroverted 子宮後傾

uterus perforation 子宮穿孔

uterus repture 子宮破裂

vagina 陰道

vaginal discharge 陰道排泌

vaginal examination 陰道檢查

vaginal examination, speculum 陰道窺器檢查

vaginitis 陰道炎

vaginitis, fungal 霉菌陰道炎

vaginitis, senile 老年性陰道炎

vaginitis, trichomonas 滴蟲陰道炎

venereal disease 性病

version 胎兒轉向術

vesicovaginal fistula 膀胱陰道瘻

vulva 外陰

vulva, pruritus 外陰癢

vulvitis 外陰炎

vulvovaginitis 外陰陰道炎

11 Paediatrics 小兒科

abstinence 戒口

achondroplasia
頓骨發育不全症

acne 暗瘡，粉刺

adolescence 青年期

adrenogenital syndrome
腎上性腺綜合徵狀

albinism 白化病

alkaptonuria 黑尿病

allergic rhinitis 過敏性鼻炎
（變態反應性鼻炎）

ambiguous genitalia
性器官不明確

amoebiasis 變型蟲病

angioedema, hereditary
遺傳性血管性水腫

antenatal 出生前

appendicitis 闌尾炎

arthritis, juvenile idiopathic
幼年類風濕性關節炎

ascariasis 蛔蟲病

asphyxia neonatorum
初生兒窒息

asthma 哮喘

ataxia 平衡失調

atrial septal defect
心房間隔缺損

autism 不受外界影響的自律性

BCG 卡介苗

battered child syndrome
虐兒綜合症

biliary atresia 膽管閉鎖

bilirubin 膽紅質

bilirubin, conjugated
接合後膽紅質

bilirubin, unconjugated
未接合膽紅質

birth injury 出生創傷

bone marrow biopsy
骨髓活組織檢驗

booster injection 加強輔助注射

branchial cyst 鰓囊

branchial fistula 鰓瘻管

bronchitis 支氣管炎

bronchiolitis 細微支氣管炎

bronchopulmonary dysplasia
肺氣管形態失常

cerebral palsy 大腦性癱瘓

cheilosis 唇乾裂

chickenpox 水痘

child abuse 虐待兒童

choledochal cyst 膽管囊腫

chorea 舞蹈病

chromosome 染色體

chronic granulimatous disease
慢性肉芽生長性疾病

cleft lip 裂唇

cleft palate 裂腭

clonus 陣攣

coarctation of aorta
主動脈縮窄

coeliac disease 粥樣瀉

common variable
immunodeficiency
常見變異性免疫力缺乏

congenital 先天性

congenital atresia of intestine
先天性小腸閉鎖

congenital megacolon
(Hirschsprung's disease)
先天性巨結腸

convulsion 抽搐 (抽筋)

convulsion, febrile 發熱性抽搐

cremasteric reflex 提睪反射

cretinism 呆小症

croup 哮吼

cryptorchidism 隱睪病

cyanosis 發紫，發紺

cystic fibrosis 中性結締組織
增生

day care centre 日間托兒中心

development 發育

dermatomyositis, juvenile
幼年皮肌炎

dextrocardia 右位心

diabetes insipidus 尿崩症

diabetes mellitus 糖尿病

diagnosis, prenatal 產前診斷

diphtheria 白喉

dominant gene 顯性基因

Down syndrome 唐氏綜合症

dwarfism 侏儒病

eczema 濕疹

encephalitis 腦炎

encephalocele 腦外突

enuresis 遺尿

epiglottities

epilepsy 癲癇 (發羊吊)

epilepsy, grand mal
  癲癇大發作

epilepsy, petit mal 癲癇小發作

epispadias 尿道上裂

exchange transfusion
  交替輸血法

exomphalos 臍突逸

exstrophy of bladder 膀胱外翻

fontanelle 囟，囟門

gargoylism 脂肪鞭骨營養不良

gene 基因 (遺傳因子)

gene, dominant 顯性基因

gene, recessive 隱性基因

genetic counselling 遺傳輔導

giardiasis 鞭毛蟲病

glomerulonephritis, acute
  急性腎小球性腎炎

glomerulonephritis, chronic
  慢性腎小球性腎炎

glucose-6-phosplate
  dehydrogenase deficiency
  6-磷酸葡萄糖脫氫酶缺乏症

growth 生長

growth retardation 生長遲緩

haemangioma 血管瘤

haemolytic disease of the
  newborn 初生血溶解病

haemophilia, hemophilia
  血友病

haemorrhage, intraventricular
  胸室出血

hereditary 遺傳

hereditary spherocytosis
  遺傳性球形紅細胞病

hermaphrodite 陰陽人

hernia 疝

hernia, diaphragmatic
  橫隔膜疝

hernia, inguinal 腹股溝疝

hernia, umbilical 臍疝

histiocytosis, Langerhan's cell 浪氏組織細胞增生

homocystinuria 高胱氨酸尿

hookworm 鈎蟲

hyaline membrane disease 透明膜病

hydrocele 鞘膜積水 (水囊腫)

hydrocephalus 腦積水

hyperactive 過度活躍

hypospadias 尿道下裂

icterus (jaundice) 黃疸

icterus, kern 核質性黃疸

ileus 腸梗阻

ileus, mechanical 機械性腸梗阻

ileus, meconium 胎糞性腸梗阻

ileus, paralytic 麻痹性腸梗阻

immunization 免疫法

immunologic deficiency 免疫缺乏

imperforate anus 肛門閉鎖

impetigo 膿疱病

inborn error of metabolism 先天性新陳代謝出錯

infantile autism 小兒自閉症

infantile spasm 小兒痙攣

infection 感染，傳染

infection, bacterial 細菌感染

infection, fungal 霉菌感染

infection, mycotic 黴菌感染

infection, viral 過濾性病菌感染

intersex 雌雄間體

intussusception 腸套疊 (套腸)

jaundice (icterus) 黃疸

jaundice, physiological 生理性黃疸

kernicterus 腦核黃疸

Klinefelter's syndrome 男性不全綜合徵狀

labour, labor 分娩，生產

lead poisoning 鉛中毒

liver function test 肝功能檢驗

local 局部性

low birth weight 出生低體重

lumbar puncture 腰椎穿刺

malaria 瘧疾

malnutrition 營養不良

malrotation of intestine 腸旋轉異常

measles 麻疹

Meckel's diverticulum 迴腸憩室

medulloblastoma 髓母細胞瘤

meningitis 腦膜炎

meningocele 腦膜外突

meningomyelocele
脊髓脊膜外突

mental retardation
智力發展遲緩 (弱智)

mesenteric lymphadenitis
腸系膜淋巴腺炎

mongolian spot 胎斑

moulding, molding 兒頭順變

mumps 流行性腮腺炎 (痄腮)

muscular dystrophy
肌肉增長不良

myoclonic 肌陣攣

myotonic 肌強直

neonatal 新生期

neonatal hepatitis 新生肝炎

nephritic syndrome
腎炎綜合症

nephroblastoma 腎胚胎癌

nephrotic syndrome
腎變病綜合症

neuroblastoma 神經母細胞癌

neurofibromatosis 神經纖維瘤

new-born 新生嬰兒

oesophageal atresia 食管閉鎖

omphalocele 臍膨突

osteogenic sarcoma 骨性肉瘤

osteomyelitis 骨髓炎

otitis media 中耳炎

pallor 蒼白

patent ductus arteriosus
動脈導管不閉症

pertussis 百日咳

phenylketonuria 尿酮苯

phimosis 包莖

pilonidal cyst 毛窩囊

pilonidal sinus 毛窩竇

pneumococcus 肺炎球菌

pneumonia 肺炎

pneumonia, lobar 肺葉炎

poliomyelitis 脊髓灰質炎
(小兒麻痹症)

polycystic kidney 多囊腎

polycystic liver 多囊肝

polyp (juvenile) 息肉 (幼年性)

postnasal drip 鼻後滴涕

pre-implantation genetic
diagnsois
殖前基因診斷

preauricular sinus 耳前竇

premature 早產

proteinuria 蛋白尿

psoriasis 銀屑病 (牛皮癬)

puberty 發育期

purpura 瘀斑

pyloric stenosis 幽門狹窄

rabies 瘋狗症

rash 疹

recessive gene 隱性基因

retinopathy of premaurity
早熟性視網膜病變

Rh incompatibility
血因素不相配

rheumatic fever 風濕性熱

rickets 佝僂病 (軟骨病)

roundworm 蛔蟲

rubella 風疹 (德國麻疹)

Salmonella 傷寒菌

scabies 疥瘡

scald 燙傷

scarlet fever 猩紅熱

scurvy 壞血症

septicaemia, septicemia 血中毒

serum bilirubin 血清膽紅素

severe combined immunodeficiency
嚴重混合免疫力不足

sex-linked hereditary
性相連遺傳

sickle cell anaemia
鐮狀細胞性貧血

smallpox 天花

spasm 痙攣 (抽筋)

speech defect 語言缺陷

spina bifida 脊柱裂

staphylococcus 葡萄球菌

strabismus 斜眼 (鬥雞眼)

streptococcus 鏈球菌

suture, bone 骨縫

syndactyly 併指 (趾) 畸形

syndrome, immotile cilia
纖毛不動徵候群

taeniasis 條蟲病

talipes equinovarus
馬蹄內翻足

teratoma 畸胎瘤

tetanus 破傷風

thalassaemia
地中海形血紅素貧血

thymus gland 胸腺

thyroglossal cyst 甲狀腺舌囊

tick 蝨

tinea 癬

tongue-tie 結舌

torticollis 斜頸

tracheo-oesophageal fistula
氣管食道瘻

tracheobronchitis
氣管支氣管炎

trichinosis 旋毛蟲病，蟠蟲病

tuberous sclerosis
管狀硬化

Turner's syndrome
女性不全綜合徵狀

ultraviolet light therapy
紫外光療法

urachal cyst 臍尿管囊腫

urachus 臍尿管

urachus, patent 臍尿管不閉

urticaria 蕁麻疹 (風疹塊)

vaccination 防疫注射

venepuncture
靜脈穿刺術 (抽血)

ventricular septal defect
心室間隔缺損

vitelline duct 卵黃管

vitiligo 白斑 (白蝕)

volvulus 腸扭轉

vomiting 嘔吐

vomiting, projectile
射出性嘔吐

wart 疣

Wilms' tumour 腎胚胎癌

Wiskott-Aldrich syndrome
維斯高亞理綜合症

X-linked
agammaglobulinaemia
X 連接球蛋白缺乏症

12 Haematological and Lymphatic System
血液與淋巴系統

acquired immunodeficiency
syndrome (AIDS) 後天性免
疫缺乏綜合症 (愛滋病)

agranulocytosis
粒白血細胞缺乏症

albumin 清蛋白

amyloidosis 澱粉樣變性

anaemia, anemia 貧血

anaemia, aplastic
缺繁殖性貧血
(再造不良性貧血)

anaemia, folate-deficiency
缺葉酸貧血

anaemia, haemolytic
溶血性貧血

anaemia, hypochromic
低色紅細胞性貧血

anaemia, iron-deficiency
缺鐵性貧血

anaemia, megaloblastic
巨紅母細胞性貧血

anaemia, microcytic
小紅細胞性貧血

anaemia, sickle cell
鐮狀細胞貧血

anaemia, vitamin B12
deficiency
缺維生素 B12 貧血

antibody 抗體

anticoagulation 防止凝血

antigen 抗原

antithrombin 抗凝血酶

autoantibody 自身抗體

biopsy 活組織檢驗

bleeding time 流血時間

blood 血液

blood group 血型

blood typing and cross match
血型分類與相對配血

bone marrow 骨髓

bone marrow biopsy
骨髓活組織檢驗

bone marrow transplant
(BMT) 骨髓移植

BMT, autologous
自體骨髓移植

BMT, allogeneic 異體骨髓移植

BMT, unrelated donor
無血緣骨髓移植

carbon monoxide poisoning
一氧化碳中毒

chemotherapy 藥物治療

chyle 乳糜

cisterna chyli 乳糜池

clotting time 凝血時間

coagulation 血凝固

coagulation defect 凝血不良

coagulation factor 凝血因素

coagulation test 凝血試驗

complete blood count (CBC)
血細胞數量檢查

congenital 先天性

Coombs' test 血抗體化驗

cyanosis 發紫，發紺

differential count
白血細胞分類計數

ecchymosis 瘀斑

eosinophilia
嗜伊紅白血細胞增多

erythropoiesis 紅細胞生成

essential thrombocythaemia
原發性血小板增多

fibrin 纖維蛋白

fibrinolysis 纖維蛋白溶解

fragility 脆性

fresh frozen plasma
新鮮冷藏血漿

fungal infection 真菌感染

genetic counselling 遺傳學輔導

genetics 遺傳學

glucose 6-phosphate
dehydrogenase deficiency
6-磷酸葡萄糖脱氫酶缺乏症

haemachromatosis, hemachromatosis
血色沉着病

haematocrit, hematocrit
紅血細胞壓積量

haematologist, hematologist
血液學家

haematology, hematology
血液學

haematopoietic growth factor
血細胞增長激素

haematopoietic stem cell transplant 血幹細胞移植

haematuria, hematuria 血尿

haemoglobin (HgB), hemoglobin 血紅素

haemoglobin, carboxy
一氧化碳血紅素

haemoglobin, met 變性血紅素

haemoglboin, oxy 氧合血紅素

haemoglobin level 血紅素濃度

haemoglobinuria, hemoglobinuria 血紅素尿

haemoglobinuria, paroxysmal nocturnal
陣發性夜間血紅素尿

haemolysis, hemolysis
血球溶解

haemophilia, hemophilia
血友病

haemorrhage, hemorrhage
出血

haemoglobin H disease
H-血紅素病

haemosiderin, hemosiderin
血黃素

haemosiderosis, hemosiderosis
血黃素沉積病

haptoglobin 親血色球蛋白

hepatomegaly 肝大

hereditary 遺傳

histiocytosis 組織細胞增多病

Hodgkin's lymphoma
何杰金氏淋巴癌

human immunodeficiency virus (HIV) 破壞免疫病毒
(愛滋病毒)

immune thrombocytopenic purpur 免疫性血少板減少

immunity 免疫

immunoglobulin 免疫球蛋白

infectious mononucleosis
傳染性單核細胞增多症

jaundice (icterus) 黃疸

leucocyte 白血細胞

leucocytosis 白血細胞增多

leucopenia 白血細胞減少

leucopheresis 白血球減除術

leukaemia, leukemia
白血細胞癌

leukaemia, acute granulocytic
急性粒白血細胞癌

leukaemia, acute lymphocytic
急性淋巴白血細胞癌

leukaemia, chronic granulocytic 慢性粒白血細胞癌

leukaemia, chronic lymphocytic
慢性淋巴白血細胞癌

leukaemia, monocytic
單核白血細胞癌

lymph 淋巴液

lymph node 淋巴結

lymphadenitis 淋巴結炎

lymphadenopathy 淋巴結病

lymphatic 淋巴系統

lymphatic gland 淋巴腺

lymphatic system 淋巴系統

lymphatic vessel 淋巴管

lymphocele 淋巴囊腫

lymphocyte 淋巴細胞

lymphoedema 淋巴水腫

lymphogram 淋巴 X 光造影

lymphoma 淋巴癌

macrophage 巨噬細胞

malaria 瘧疾

megakaryocyte 巨核細胞

metabolic disorder
新陳代謝異常

metabolism 新陳代謝

multiple myeloma
多發性骨髓癌

myelodysplasia 骨髓異變

myelofibrosis 骨髓纖維化

myoglobinuria 肌球蛋白尿

neutropenia 中性白細胞減少

non-Hodgkin's lymphoma
非何杰金氏淋巴癌

neutropenic infection
低中細胞感染

pallor 蒼白

parasite 寄生蟲

peripheral smear
血抹片 (檢查)

peripheral stem cell 血幹細胞

pernicious anaemia 惡性貧血

petechia 瘀點

plasmacytoma 漿細胞癌

plasmaphaeresis, plasmapheresis 血漿隔除術
血漿減除術

platelet 血小板

polycythaemia, polycythemia
紅血細胞增多

polycythaemia vera
真性紅血細胞增多

porphyria 紫質沉著病

primary 原發，第一期

prothrombin time
凝血酵素原時間

purpura 紫癜

radioactive 放射性

radioactive isotope
放射性同位素

radiotherapy 放射治療

red blood cell (RBC)
紅血細胞 (紅血球)

red cell count 紅血細胞數量

remission 緩解

reticulo-endothelial system
網狀內皮系統

reticulocyte count
網狀紅血細胞數量

serum 血清

spectrophotometry 分光測定法

splenectomy 脾切除術

splenomegaly 脾大

synthesis 合成

thalassaemia
地中海形血紅素貧血

thoracic duct 淋巴主導管

thrombocytopenia
血小板減少病

transfusion 輸血

transfusion, exchange
交替輸血法

ulceration 潰瘍

umbilical cored blood
transplant 臍帶血移植

white blood cell (WBC)
白血細胞 (白血球)

white blood cell, basophil
嗜鹼白血細胞

white blood cell, eosinophil
嗜伊紅白血細胞

white blood cell, lymphocyte
淋巴白血細胞

white blood cell, monocyte
單核白血細胞

white blood cell, plasma cell
血漿細胞

white blood cell, polymorph
neutrophil 嗜中性白血細胞

white cell count 白血細胞數量

13 Neurological System
神經系統

abscess, spinal 脊椎膿瘍

abscess, subdural 硬膜下膿瘍

acoustic neuroma 聽覺神經瘤

acute brachial neuritis 急性臂神經炎

acute compression 急性壓迫性脊髓病

acute disseminated encephalomyelitis 急性麥芽醣欠損症

acute haemorrhagic leucoencephalitis 急性出血性白盾腦炎

acute thrombolysis 急性血栓溶解治療

addiction 上癮

agnosia 失知 (病)

Alzheimer's disease 阿氏癡呆症

amaurosis fugax 短暫性黑蒙 (病)

amblyopia 弱視

amnesia 失憶，失憶病

amyotrophic lateral sclerosis 肌萎縮性側索硬化症

analgesic 止痛藥

analgic 失痛 (病)

angioma 血管瘤

ankylosing spondylitis 關節硬化性脊椎炎

anosmia 嗅覺喪失

anticoagulation 抗凝血藥物

anticonvulsant 抗抽搐藥

antidepressant 抗抑鬱藥

antiepileptic drugs 抗癲癇藥

antiplatelet agents 抗血小皮劑

aphasia 失語 (病)

aphonia 失音 (病)

apraxia 失用 (病)

arachnoid 蛛網膜

argyll Robertson pupil 阿吉爾-羅伯森氏瞳孔

arnold-chiari malformation 先天性小腦廷髓下疝畸形

arteriosclerotic dementia 動脈硬化性痴呆

arteriosclerotic parkinsonism 動脈硬化性帕金森氏綜合症

arteriovenous malformation 動靜脈畸形

arteritis 動脈炎

astrocytoma 星形細胞瘤

ataxia 協調缺失 (病)

athetoid 指痙

athetosis 手足徐動病

atlantoaxial dislocation 寰樞脱位

auditory 聽覺

autonomic nervous system 自主神經系統

autonomic neuropathy 自主神經病

axonotmesis 軸突斷裂

basal ganglia 基底神經節

Bell's palsy 面神經痲痺症

belpharospasm 瞼痙攣

benign essential tremor 良性原發性震顫

benign intracranial hypertension 良性顱內高壓

benign paroxysmal positional vertigo 良性陣發性位置性眩暈

berry aneurysm 顱內漿果狀動脈瘤

bitemporal hemianopia 雙顳側偏盲

blood brain barrier 血腦屏障

botulinum toxin 肉毒毒素

brain concussion 腦震盪

brain contusion 腦撞傷

brain death 腦死亡

brain laceration 腦裂傷

brain scan 放射性腦掃描

brain stem 腦干

brainstem auditory evoked potentials 腦幹聽覺誘發電位檢查

bulbar palsy 廷髓痲痺

burr hole 頭骨鑽孔

carcinomatous 癌性腦膜轉移

carotid endarterectomy
頸動脈內膜剝離術

cauda equina 脊髓尾

cavernous sinus aneurysm
海綿竇動脈瘤

cavernous sinus thrombosis
海綿靜脈竇血栓塞

central nervous system
中樞神經系統

central pontine myelinolysis
橋腦中央脱髓鞘症

cerebello-pontine angle lesion
小腦—橋腦角病變

cerebellum 小腦

cerebral 大腦的

cerebral abscess 大腦膿腫

cerebral angiography
腦血管造影術

cerebral artery 大腦動脈

cerebral artery aneurysm
大腦動脈瘤 (樣膨大)

cerebral cortex 大腦皮層

cerebral embolism 腦栓子

cerebral haemorrhage
(大) 腦出血

cerebral hemisphere 大腦半球

cerebral infarction
大腦梗塞壞死

cerebral ischaemia 大腦缺血

cerebral lymphoma
大腦淋巴瘤

cerebral oedema 腦水腫

cerebral palsy 大腦性癱瘓

cerebral spinal fluid 脊髓液

cerebral thrombosis 腦血栓塞

cerebral tumor 大腦腫瘤

cerebral vascular accident
中風

cerebral venous thrombosis
大腦靜脈血栓

cerebrovascular disease 腦血
管病，腦血管疾病

cerebrum 大腦

cervical myelopthy 頸脊髓病

cervical rib 頸肋

cervical spondylotic
myelopathy 頸椎脊髓病

charcot's joint 神經性關節病

chorea 舞蹈病

cluster headache 叢集性頭痛，
叢發性頭痛

cogwheel rigidity 齒輪樣僵硬

coma 昏迷

communicating
hydrocephalus
交通性腦積水

compression 壓迫

concussion 震盪

conduction 傳導

coning (herniation of brain)大腦脫垂 (大腦內癌)

contracture 攣縮

contusion 挫傷

convulsion 抽搐 (抽筋)

co-ordination 協調

cordotomy 脊椎柱切斷術

cortical blindness 腦皮層盲

corticosteroid 腎上腺皮層素

cranial nerve 顱神經

cranial nerve I - olfactory 顱神經 I - 嗅覺神經

cranial nerve II - optic 顱神經 II - 視覺神經

cranial nerve III - oculomotor 顱神經 III - 眼活動神經

cranial nerve IV - trochlear 顱神經 IV - 滑輪神經

cranial nerve V - trigeminal 顱神經 V - 三叉神經

cranial nerve VI - abducent 顱神經 VI - 外展神經

cranial nerve VII - facial 顱神經 VII - 面神經

cranial nerve VIII - vestibular; cochlear 顱神經 VIII - 平衡神經 ；聽覺神經

cranial nerve IX - glossopharyngeal 顱神經 IX - 舌咽神經

cranial nerve X - vagus 顱神經 X - 迷走神經

cranial nerve XI - accessory 顱神經 XI - 附屬神經

cranial nerve XII - hypoglossal 顱神經 XII - 舌下神經

craniectomy 顱骨切除術

craniopharyngioma 顱咽管瘤

craniotomy 顱骨切開術

cryptococcal meningitis 隱球菌腦膜炎

cyclosporiin 環孢靈

cysticercosis 囊蟲病

cytomegalovirus 巨噬細胞病毒，巨細胞病毒

deaf 聾

déjà vu 似曾相識感覺

degenerative 退化性脊髓病

dementia 痴呆

dementia, senile 老年性痴呆

demyelination 脫髓鞘性脊髓病

depression 抑鬱

dermatome 皮神經區

dermatomyositis 皮肌炎

diplopia 複視

dizziness 頭暈

drowsy 神智不清

dura mater 硬腦脊膜

dysarthria 發音困難

dyskinesia 運動障礙

dyskinesia, tardive 遲發性運動
失能

dyslexia 誦讀困難

dysphonia 發音困難

dystonia 張力障礙

edinger-westphal nucleus 動眼
神經副核

electroconvulsive therapy
(ECT) 電痙攣療法

electroencephalogram (EEG)
腦電圖

electromyogram (EMG)
肌電圖

encephalitis 腦炎

encephalitis, viral
過濾性病毒腦炎

encephalopathy 腦病

ependymoma 室管膜瘤

epidural 硬膜外

epidural anaesthesia
硬膜外麻醉

epidural haematoma
硬膜外血腫

epilepsy 癲癇 (發羊吊)

epilepsy, grand-mal
癲癇大發作

epilepsy, petit-mal 癲癇小發作

evoked potential 誘發電位

extradural haematoma
硬膜外血腫

flaccid 弛緩

focal seizure 局部性癲癇

foot-drop 足下垂

foramen magnum 枕骨大孔

frontal lobe 額葉

ganglion 神經節

ganglion, stellate 星狀神經節

giddiness 眩暈

glasgow coma scale 格拉斯哥
氏昏迷指數表

glioblastoma 成膠質細胞瘤

glioma 神經膠質瘤

grasp reflex 握持反射

Guillain-Barré syndrome
急性周神經炎

haematoma, hematoma
血腫

haemophilus influenzae 流搆
嗜血桿菌腦膜炎

hallucination 幻覺

headache 頭痛

headache, frontal 額頭痛

headache, migraine 偏頭痛

headache, tension 緊張頭痛

hemianopia 偏盲

hemiballismus 偏身顫搐

hemifacial spasm
偏側面肌痙攣

hemiparesis 輕偏癱

hemiplegia 偏癱

hereditary 遺傳

homonymous hemianopia
同側偏盲

Horner's syndrome
頸交感神經麻痹綜合徵狀

hydrocephalus 腦積水

hysteria 協識脫離 (癔病)

incontinence 失禁

infarction 梗塞壞死

infection 感染性脊髓病

interferon 干擾素

intention tremor 意向性震顫

intermittent porphyria
間歇性比咯紫質沈著症

intervertebral disc 椎間盤

intoxication 中毒 (醉酒)

intracranial 顱內

intracranial pressure 顱內壓

irradiation 放射／輻射性
脊髓病

ischaemic stroke 缺血性中風

kuru 新幾內亞震顫病

laminectomy 椎盤切除術

lethargy 無精打采，懶散

loss of consciousness 喪失知覺

lower motor neuron
下運動神經元

lumbar disc lesion
腰椎間盤病變

lumbar plexus 腰神經叢

lumbar puncture 腰椎穿刺

medulloblastoma
成神經管細胞瘤

Meniere's disease 耳水不平衡

meninges 腦脊膜

meningioma 腦膜瘤

meningococcal 流行性腦膜炎

meningitis 腦膜炎

meningomyelocele
脊髓脊膜外突

meralgia paraesthetica
感覺異常性股痛

metabolic disorder
新陳代謝失調

metastasis（癌）轉移

migraine 偏頭痛

motor neuron 運動神經元

motor neuron disease
運動神經元疾病

MRI scanning 核磁共振掃描

multi-system atrophy (MSA)
多系統萎縮

multiple sclerosis 多發性硬化

muscular dystrophy
肌肉增長不良

myasthenia gravis 重性肌無力

myasthenic syndrome
肌無力綜合症

myelitis 脊髓炎

myelocele 脊髓突出

myelogram 脊髓造影

myelomeningocoele
脊髓脊膜突出

myelopathy 脊髓疾病

myoclonus 肌陣攣病

myopathy 肌病

myositis 肌炎

myositis ossificans 化朋性肌炎

narcolepsy 發作性睡病

neck stiffness 頸僵硬

neoplastic 腫瘤性脊髓病

nerve 神經

nerve conduction studies
神經傳導檢查

nerve root 神經根

neuralgia 神經痛

neurapraxia
神經失用症（機能性麻痺）

neuritis 神經炎

neuropathic bladder 神經性膀
胱功能障礙

neurofibromatosis
神經纖維瘤病

neuroma 神經瘤

neuroma, acoustic 聽覺神經瘤

neuropathy 神經病

neurosyphilis 神經梅毒

numbness 麻木

nystagmus 眼球震顫

occipital cortex 枕葉皮層

oligodendroglioma
少突膠質細胞瘤

ophthalmoplegia 眼肌麻痺

optic atrophy 視萎縮

optic neuritis 視神經炎

Paget's disease 變形性骨炎

pain clinic 痛症科診所

palsy 癱瘓

palsy, Bell's 外周臉神經癱瘓

papilloedema, papilledema
視神經乳頭體水腫

paralysis 癱瘓 (麻痹)

paraneoplastic 腫瘤副增生性
脊髓病

paraplegia 下肢癱瘓，截瘓

parasympathetic nerve
副交感神經

paresis 輕癱

parietal lobe 頂葉

Parkinsonism 帕金遜臨床表徵

Parkinson's disease 帕金遜病

Parkinson-plus syndrome
非典型帕金遜綜合徵

peripheral nervous system
外周神經系統

pia mater 軟腦膜

pituitary 腦垂體

pituitary adenoma 垂體腺瘤

plexus 神經叢

plexus, brachial 臂神經叢

pneumococcal 肺炎球菌腦膜炎

poliomyelitis
脊髓灰質炎 (小兒麻痹症)

polyarteritis nodosa 結節性多
動脈炎

polymyositis 多肌炎

pontine haemorrhage
橋腦出血

port-wine stain
焰色痣 (葡萄酒色痣)

posterior communicating
artery aneurysm
後交通／聯絡動脈動脈瘤，
後大腦動脈交通枝動脈瘤

post-immunization
encephalomyelitis

post-infectious
encephalomyelitis

proptosis 眼球突出

pseudobulbar palsy
假性球麻痹

pseudo-parkinsonism
假性帕金森氏綜合症

pseudo-seizure 假性癲癇發作

pseudobulbar palsy 假性廷腦
麻痹

ptosis 眼瞼下垂

pyogenic 化膿性腦膜炎

pyramidal sign 錐體徵象

radiation myeolopthy
放射性脊髓病

radiosurgery 放射線聚焦治療

reflex 反射 (作用)

reflex, corneal 角膜反射

reflex, cough 咳嗽反射

reflex, gag 引吐反射

reflex, pupil 瞳孔反射

reflex, sucking 吸吮反射

retinal artery occlusion 視網膜動脈阻塞

retrobulbar neuritis 球後視神經炎

rhizotomy 脊神經根切斷術

rigid 僵硬

Romberg's test 閉目難立試驗

sacral plexus 骶神經叢

sciatica 坐骨神經痛

sedative 鎮靜劑

seizure 癲癇

sensation 感覺

sexual dysfunction 性功能障礙

skull 頭顱

skull fracture 頭顱骨折

skull fracture, depressed 頭顱凹陷骨折

sjogren's syndrome 乾燥症候群

somatosensory 體覺

spasm 痙攣(抽筋)

spastic 痙攣性

spastic paraplegia 痙攣性截癱

spina bifida 脊柱裂

spinal cord 脊髓

spinal cord disorders 脊髓疾病

spinothalamic tract 脊髓丘腦束

spina bifida 脊柱裂

spinal muscular atrophy 脊髓性肌肉萎縮症

status epilepticus 癲癇連續狀態

stenosis 狹窄

stereotactic surgery 立體定向手術

stereotaxic surgery 立體定位手術

stimulant 興奮劑，刺激藥

streptococcus suis 瑞士鏈球菌腦膜炎

subarachnoid haemorrhage 蛛網膜下出血

subdural haematoma 硬膜下血腫

sympathectomy 交感神經切斷術

sympathetic nerve 交感神經

syncope 暈厥

syringomyelia 脊髓空洞症

systemic lupus erythermatosis 紅斑狼瘡

tabes dorsalis 脊髓梅毒

tetanus 破傷風

thoracic outlet syndrome
　胸廓出口綜合症

thymectomy 胸腺切除術

thymoma 胸腺瘤

tic douloureux
　抽搐性三叉神經痛

tranquillizer 安定藥

transient ischaemic attack
　(TIA) 短暫性腦缺血

transverse myelitis
　橫貫性脊髓炎

trauma 創傷性脊髓病

tremor 震顫

trigeminal neuralgia
　三叉神經痛

trismus 牙關緊閉

unconscious 昏迷 (不省人事)

upper motor neurone lesion
　上位運動神經元病灶

vascular 缺血性性脊髓病

vascular dementia
　血管性失智症

venous sinus 靜脈竇

ventricle 腦室

vertebral basilar ischaemia
　椎基底動脈供血不足

vestibular neuronitis
　前庭神經炎

vertigo 眩暈 (天旋地轉)

viral meningitis 病毒性腦炎

vision 視覺 (視力)

visual acuity 視力敏度

visual field 視野

visual pathway 視覺傳遞路徑

whiplash injury 馬鞭式創傷

14 Musculo-Skeletal System
肌胳系統

10-second test 10秒測試

abduction 外展

acetabulum 髖臼

abscess, cold 無熱膿腫

achilles tendon 腳跟鍵／阿奇里斯腱

achilles tendonitis 腳跟腱炎／阿基氏腱肌腱炎

achondroplasia 先天性頓骨發育不全

acromion 肩峯

adduction 內收

adhesive capsulitis 黏連性關節囊炎（五十肩）

alar ligament 翼狀韌帶

allograft 同種異體移植物

amputation 切除術

amputation, below knee 膝下切除術

amputation, forequarter 上肢切除術

amputation, hindquarter 下肢切除術

ankylosing spondylitis 關節硬化性脊椎炎

ankylosis 關節硬化

ankylosis, bony 骨節性關節硬化

ankylosis, fibrous 纖維性關節硬化

annulus fibrosus 椎間盤纖維環

anteflexion 前屈

anterior longitudinal ligament 前縱韌帶

anterior spinal fusin 前路椎體融合術

anteversion 前傾

aponeurosis 腱膜

arm 臂

anteriovenous malformation 動靜脉瘻

artery 動脈

arthritis 關節炎

arthritis, gonococcal 淋病性關節炎

arthritis, gouty 痛風性關節炎

arthritis, haemophilic 血友病性關節炎

arthritis, infectious 感染性關節炎

arthritis, psoriatic 牛皮癬性關節炎

arthritis, pyogenic 膿毒性關節炎

arthritis, rheumatoid 風濕性關節炎

arthritis, suppurative 化膿性關節炎

arthritis, septic 關節穿刺術

arthritis, tuberculous 結核性關節炎

arthrodesis 關節固定術

arthrodesis, triple 三重關節固定術

arthrography 關節 **X** 光造影

arthroplasty 關節造形術

arthroplasty, excision 切除性關節整形術

arthroplasty, partial replacement 局部關節代換術

arthroplasty, total replacement 全關節代換術

arthroscopy 關節鏡檢查

arthrotomy 關節切開術

articulation 關節聯接

atlantoaxial instability 寰樞椎關節不穩

atrophy 萎縮

atrophy, Sudeck's 外傷急性骨萎縮

autograft 自體移植

avascular necrosis 絕血性壞死

avulsion 撕除

axonotmesis 神經軸索斷傷

biopsy 活組織檢驗

bipolar arthroplasty 雙極關節置換

bone 骨

bone, accessory 附骨

bone, cancellous 海綿質骨

bone, carpal 腕骨

bone, clavicle 鎖骨

bone, femur 股骨

bone, fibula 腓骨

bone, flat 扁骨

bone, humerus 肱骨

bone, iliac 髂骨

bone, marble 大理石骨硬化病

bone, metacarpal 掌骨

bone, metatarsal 跖骨

bone, pelvis 骨盆

bone, phalange 指(趾)骨

bone, pubis 恥骨

bone, radius 橈骨

bone, rib 肋骨

bone, scaphoid 舟狀骨

bone, scapula 肩胛骨

bone, sesamoid 種子狀骨

bone, sternum 胸骨

bone, tarsal 跗骨

bone, tibia 脛骨

bone, ulna 尺骨

bone bank 骨庫

bone cement 骨粘固粉

bone cortex 皮質骨

bone cyst 骨囊腫

bone marrow 骨髓

bone mineral density (BMD)
骨骼物質密度／骨密度

bone necrosis 骨壞死

bone scan 骨骼掃描

bone shaft 骨幹

boutonniere deformity 鈕扣孔
式變形

bow legs 弓形腿

brace 支具／支架／梏具

brachial plexus 臂神經叢

bucket handle tear 桶柄式撕裂

bumper fracture 車撞骨折

bunion 骱囊尖腫

bunionectomy 骱囊尖腫切除術

burn 燒傷

bursa 滑液囊

bursitis 滑囊炎

calcification 鈣化

calcitonin 降鈣素

calf 腓

callus 胼胝，骨痂(接骨質)

callosity 胼胝／雞眼

carpal tunnel syndrome
腕管綜合症

carpus 腕

cartilage 輭骨

cast-brace 石膏腳規

cerebral palsy 大腦性癱瘓

cervical spondylotic myelopathy (CSM) 頸椎脊髓病

cervical spondylotic radiculopathy 頸椎退化性神經根病變

Charcot's disease 神經原性關節病

Charcot's joint 神經原性關節

chondroblastoma 成軟骨細胞瘤

chondrocalcinosis 軟骨鈣化症

chondrolysis 軟骨溶解

chondroma 軟骨瘤

chondromalacia 軟骨軟化

chondromalacia, patellae 膝蓋骨軟化

chondromatosis 軟骨瘤病

chondromyxoid fibroma 軟骨粘液纖維瘤

chondrosarcoma 軟骨肉瘤

chordoma 脊索瘤

chymopapain 木瓜凝乳蛋白酶／木瓜酵素

claw-hand 爪形手

clawed toe 爪形趾

club foot 馬蹄內翻足

computer tomography 電腦輔助手術 (骨科)

condyle 髁

congenital dislocation 先天性關節脱位

congenital dislocation of hip 先天性髖關節脱位

contracture 攣縮

COX 2 inhibitor 環氧化酶二 (COX-2) 抑制劑

cryotherapy 冷凍治療

cubitus valgus 肘外翻

cubitus varus 肘內翻

curette 刮匙

curly toe 捲縮趾

currettage 刮除術

cyst 水囊，囊腫

cyst, Baker's 膝部囊腫

cyst, meniscus 半月板囊腫

dactylitis 指 (趾) 炎

de Quervain's disease 痛性腕腱鞘炎

debridement 清創術

decompression 減壓

deep vein thrombosis 深位靜脈栓塞

deformity 變形

deformity, boutonniere 鈕孔狀變形

deformity, gunstock 槍托狀變形

deformity, swan neck
鵝頸狀變形

degenerative disc disease (DDD) 退行椎間板病變／退化性椎間盤疾病

desmoid tumour 硬纖維瘤

diaphysis 骨幹

disarticulation 關節斷離術

disc 盤

disc, intervertebral 椎間盤

discitis 椎間盤炎

dislocation 脫位

dislocation, habitual 慣性脫位

dislocation, perilunate
半月骨周圍脫位

dislocation, permanent
永久性脫位

dislocation, recurrent
再發性脫位

dislocation, voluntary
隨意性脫位

drawer test 抽屜試驗

drop, foot 足下垂

drop, wrist 腕下垂

Dupuytren's contracture
掌攣縮病

dwarf 侏儒

dwarfism 侏儒病

dynamic hip screw (DHS) 動力髖螺釘

dyschondroplasia
軟骨發育不良

dysplasia 增殖不良

dysplasia, fibrous
纖維性增殖不良

dysplasia epiphysealis
骨骺增殖不良

dystrophy 增長不良

elbow 肘

elbow, tennis 網球家肘病

electromyogram (EMG)
肌電圖

enchondroma 內生軟骨瘤

eosinophilic granuloma
嗜伊紅性肉芽腫

elbow, gofer's 過爾夫球肘

elbow, pitcher's 棒球 (壘球) 投手肘

elbow, tennis 網球肘

entrapment neuropathy 外圍神經卡壓病變／慢性陷套神經病變

epicondyle 上髁

epiphyseal plate 板

epiphysis 骺

epiphysis, slipped upper femoral 上股骨骺脫離

Erb palsy Erb 氏 (臂神經叢) 麻痺

erysipeloid 類丹毒

eversion 外翻

exostosis 外生骨疣 (骨刺)

external fixator 外固定架

extension 伸直

extracorporeal shock wave therapy (ESWT) 體外衝擊波治療

fascia 闊筋膜

fasciectomy 筋膜切除術

fasciitis 筋膜炎

fasciotomy 筋膜切開術

fat 脂肪，肥胖

fat, embolism 脂肪栓塞

fenestration 開窗手術

fibroma 纖維瘤

fibromaosis 纖維瘤病

fibrosarcoma 纖維肉癌

fibrosis 纖維化

fibrositis 纖維組織炎

fibrous cortical defect 纖維性骨皮缺陷

fibrous dysplasia 纖維性增殖不良

finger 指

finger, index 食指，示指

finger, little 小指

finger, mallet 槌狀指

finger, middle 中指

finger, ring 環指，無名指

finger, trigger 扳機指

fingertip 指尖

fixation 固定術

fixation, external 外固定術

fixation, internal 內固定術

flatfoot 扁平足

flexion 屈曲

foot 足 (腳)

forearm 前臂

fracture 骨折，折斷

fracture, avulsion 撕除性骨折

fracture, Barton's (巴爾通氏) 骨折

fracture, Bennett's (貝奈特氏) 骨折

fracture, burst 破碎骨折

frafture, closed 無外傷骨折

fracture, Colles' 科勒斯氏 (橈骨下端) 骨折

fracture, comminuted 粉碎骨折

fracture, compound 複式骨折

fracture, compression 受壓性骨折

fracture, condylar 髁骨折

fracture, crack 骨裂

fracture, dislocation 脫位骨折

fracture, displaced 移位骨折

fracture, greenstick 青枝骨折

fracture, hairline 髮線形骨折

fracture, impacted 嵌入骨折

fracture, intra-articular
關節內骨折

fracture, march 行軍骨折

fracture, oblique 斜骨折

fracture, open 外傷骨折

fracture, pathologic 病變骨折

fracture, Pott's 腓骨下端骨折

**fracture, separation of
epiphysis** 骨折性骺脫離

fracture, simple 單純骨折

fracture, spiral 螺旋形骨折

fracture, stress 應力性骨折

fracture, supracondylar
髁上骨折

fracture, transverse 橫骨折

frozen joint 關節硬化

frozen shoulder 凍肩／五十肩
／肩周炎

gait 步態

ganglion 腱鞘囊腫

ganglion, compound palmar
複合性掌側囊腫

gangrene 壞疽

gangrene, gas 氣性壞疽

genu 膝

genu, recurvatum 膝反屈

genu, valgum 膝外翻

genu, varum 膝內翻

giant cell tumour 巨細胞瘤

glomus tumour 血管球瘤

goniometer 測角儀

gout 痛風

graft 移植，移植物

graft, autogenous 自體移植

graft, bone 骨移植

graft, cable 電纜式神經移植

graft, cross finger flap
鄰指皮瓣移植

graft, cross leg flap
鄰肢皮瓣移植

graft, flap 移植瓣

graft, free vascularized
血管化游離移植

graft, full-thickness skin
全層皮膚移植

graft, heterogenous 異種移植

graft, homologous
同種異體移植

graft, nerve 神經移植

graft, neurovascular island
島狀瓣神經血管移植

graft, pedicle 蒂狀移植

graft, skin 皮膚移植

graft, split thickness skin
(STSG) 表層皮膚移植

graft, tnedon 腱移植

graft, vascularized bone
血管化骨移植

granuloma pyogenicum
化膿性肉芽

growth 生長

gunshot wound 槍傷

haemangioma, hemangioma
血管瘤

haemarthrosis
關節血腫

hallux 䟛趾

hallux, rigidus 僵䟛，䟛強直

hallux, valgus 䟛外翻

hallux varus 大趾內翻／拇趾
內翻

halo 暈輪

halo, cast 暈輪石膏背夾

halo, femoral traction
暈輪股牽引

halo, jacket 暈輪背夾

halo, pelvic traction
暈輪骨盤牽引

hammer toe 鎚狀趾／錘狀趾

hand 手

hand, claw 爪形手

hand, lobster 裂手

heel 腳跟

hemiarthroplasty 半關節整形
術／半關節置換術

Horner's syndrome
頸交感神經麻痺綜合徵狀

hyperextension 伸直過度

hyperhidrosis 多汗症

hypermobility 移動性過度

hyperreflexia 反射過強

hypertrophic 增生性／肥厚性

immobilization 制動 (術)

implant 植入 (物)

incision and drainage
(I and D) 切開引流

ingrown toe-nail 趾甲內嵌

insertion 插入

internal fixation 內固定 (手術)

intervertebral disc 椎間盤

intoeing 內八字足

intramedullary nail
朋髓內釘／髓內釘

intrinsic 內在，內有

inversion 內翻

involucrum 包殼

involuntary 不隨意

ischaemia, ischemia 缺血

ischaemic contracture
 缺血性攣縮

ischaemic necrosis 缺血性壞死

isograft 卵雙生子移植

joint 關節

joint, ankle 踝關節

joint, ball and socket 球窩關節

joint, carpal 腕關節

joint, cartilage 輭骨關節

joint, Charcot's
 神經原性關節 (病)

joint, elbow 肘關節

joint, hinge 屈成關節

joint, hip 髖關節

joint, interphalangeal
 指 (趾) 骨間關節

joint, knee 膝關節

joint, midcarpal 腕中關節

joint, midtarsal 跗中關節

joint, shoulder 肩關節

joint, subtalar
 距跟關節 (踝骨下關節)

joint, wrist 腕關節

joint contracture 關節代積水

joint effusion 關節鬆弛

joint laxity 關節鬆弛

joint prosthesis 關節代換體

knee 膝

knee, knock 膝內翻

knee, housemaid's 家庭主婦膝

kyphosis 脊柱後彎

labrum 唇，緣

labrum, acetabular 髖臼緣

labrum, glenoid 盂緣

lamina 椎盤

laminectomy 椎板切開

lateral 外側

laxity 鬆弛

leprosy 痲瘋

ligament 韌帶

ligament, annular 環狀韌帶

ligament, cruciate
 (膝) 十字韌帶

ligament, deltoid 三角韌帶

ligament, plantar
 蹠側韌帶，足底韌帶

ligamentum, flavum 黃韌帶

ligamentum, teres 圓韌帶

limb 肢

limb salvage surgery 保肢手術／肢體保留手術

limp 蹣跚／跛行

locked knee 膝閉鎖

losse body 關節遊動體

lordosis 脊柱前凸

lumbar disc prolapse 腰椎間盤脱出

lumbar spondylosis 腰椎間退化病

lymphatic 淋巴系統

magnetic resonance imaging (MRI) 磁力共振造影

malignant fibrous histiocytoma 惡性纖維組織細胞瘤

malunion 連接不良

manipulation 推拿術

manual therapy 手法治療／徒手治療

medial 內側

medulla （骨）髓／髓質

meningocele 腦膜外突，脊膜外突

meniscectomy 半月板切除術

meniscus 半月板

meniscus, cyst 半月板囊腫

microsurgery 顯微外科，顯微手術

miliary tuberculosis 粟粒性結核病

minimally invasive surgery 微創 (外科) 手術

mucopolysaccharidosis 粘多糖病

muscle 肌

muscle, biceps 二頭肌

muscle, extensor 伸肌

muscle, flexor 屈肌

muscle, smooth 平滑肌

muscle, sphincter 括約肌

muscle, striated 橫紋肌

muscle, triceps 三頭肌

muscle atrophy 肌萎縮

muscular dystrophy 肌肉增長不良

musculus, beceps femoris 股二頭肌

musculus, biceps brachii 肱二頭肌

musculus, coccygeus 尾骨肌

musculus, deltoideus 三角肌

musculus, erector spinae 堅棘肌

musculus, gastrocnemius 腓腸肌

musculus, glutaeus maximus 臀大肌

musculus, latissimus dorsi 背闊肌

musculus, levator scapulae 提肩胛肌

musculus, popliteus 膕肌

musculus, pronator teres 旋前圓肌

musculus, quadratus femoris 股方肌

musculus, rectus abdominis 腹直肌

musculus, sacrospinalis 骶棘肌

musculus, scalenus anterior 前斜角肌

musculus, sternocleidomastoideus 胸鎖乳突肌

musculus, transversus abdominis 腹橫肌

musculus, trapezius 斜方肌

musculus, triceps brachii 肱三頭肌

myasthenia gravis 重性肌無力

myelogram 脊髓造影

myelography 脊髓造影術

myeloma 脊髓細胞瘤

myelomeningocele 脊髓脊膜突出

myopathy 肌病

myositis ossificans 骨化性肌炎

nail 指甲，趾甲

nailing 插釘術

navigation 導航

necrosis 壞死

necrosis, aseptic 無菌性壞死

necrosis, avascular 絕血性壞死

necrosis, fibrinoid 類纖維壞死

nerve 神經

neuralgia 神經痛

neurapraxia 神經失用症 (機能性麻痺)

neurilemmoma 神經膜瘤

neuroma 神經瘤

neuropraxia 神經失用 (機能性麻痺)

neurotmesis 神經斷傷

non-union 不連合

nucleus pulposus 椎間盤核

nutrient artery 滋養動脈

onychogryphosis 甲彎曲

open reduction and internal fixation 切開復位內固定術

origin 起端，起源

orthopaedic sports medicine 骨科運動醫

orthosis 矯形支具

Osgood-Schlatter disease 脛骨粗隆頓骨病

ossification 骨化

ossification, heterotopic 異位骨化

ossification centre 骨化中心

osteitis deformans (Paget's disease of bone) 畸形性骨炎

osteitis fibrosa cystica (von Recklinghausen's disease of bone) 纖維性囊狀骨炎

osteoarthritis 骨性關節炎

osteochondritis 骨性頓骨炎

osteochondritis dissecans 剝脫性骨軟骨炎／分割性骨軟骨炎

osteogenesis imperfecta 成骨不全

osteogenic osteoma 骨原性骨瘤

osteogenic sarcoma 骨肉癌

osteoid osteoma 骨樣骨瘤

osteolysis 骨組織化解

osteoma 骨瘤

osteomalacia 骨頓化

osteomyelitis 骨髓炎

osteomyelitis, tuberculosis 結核骨髓炎

ostenecrosis 缺血性骨壞死／骨壞死

osteopetrosis 骨石化

osteophyte 骨贅

osteoporosis 骨質疏鬆

osteosarcoma 骨肉瘤

osteosclerosis 骨硬化

osteotomy 切骨術

outtoeing 外八字足

paralysis 癱瘓（麻痺）

paraplegia 下身癱瘓，截癱

parathormone 甲狀旁腺激素

paronychia 甲溝炎

pes planus 扁平足

plantar fasciitis 足底筋膜炎

plantar wart 腳掌疣

plaster 石膏

poliomyelitis 脊髓灰質炎（小兒麻痺症）

polydactyly 多指（趾）畸形

polymyositis 多肌炎

popliteal, cyst 膕囊腫

popliteal space 膕窩

positron emission tomography (PET) 正子斷層掃描／正子造影

prolapsed intervertebral disc 椎間盤脫出

pronation 旋前

prone 俯臥

prosthesis 代換肢，代換體

pseudarthrosis 假關節

pseudogout 假痛風

pubic ramus 恥骨枝

reduction 復位 (術)

reduction, closed
　不切開回復 (術)

reduction, open 切開回復術

rehabilittion 復康

re-implant 再植 (入)

renal osteodystrophy
　腎病骨增殖不良

replantation, digital 斷指再植

replantation, limb 斷肢再植

reticulum cell sarcoma
　網狀細胞肉癌

revision arthroplasty
　關節翻修術

rhabdomyosarcoma
　橫紋肌肉癌

rheumatoid factors
　類風濕因子

rheumatoid focus 風濕病灶

rheumatoid nodule 風濕結

rib 肋骨

rickets 佝僂病 (軟骨病)

rotation 旋轉

rotation, external 外旋轉

rotation, internal 內旋轉

rotator cuff 肩袖

sarcoma 肉癌

scoliosis 脊柱側凸

scoliosis, congenital
　先天性脊柱側凸

scurvy 壞血病

sequestrum 死骨 (片)

sesamoid bone 種子狀骨

shock 休克

short-wave diathermy
　短波透熱電療法

sinus 竇

sinus tract 竇管

skeleton 骨骼

skier's thumb 滑雪者拇指

skin graft, split thickness
　表層皮膚移植

skin graft, full thickness
　全層皮膚移植

spasmodic flat foot 痙攣性平足

spina bifida 脊柱裂

spinal claudication 脊柱神經性
　歇性跛行

spinal cord 脊髓

spinal stenosis 脊管狹窄／椎管
　狹窄

spine 脊柱

spine, cervical 脊柱頸段，頸椎

spine, lumbar 脊柱腰段，腰椎

spine, sacral 脊柱骶段，骶椎

spine, thoracic 脊柱胸段，胸椎

splint 夾 (板)，梏具

spondylitis 脊椎炎

spondylolisthesis 椎骨脱位病

spondylolysis 椎骨崩解病

spondylosis
椎骨盤退化病 (椎關節黏連)

sprain 扭傷

stenosing tenovaginitis
狹窄性腱鞘炎

stiff 僵硬

strain 勞損／過勞／拉傷

subacromial bursitis 肩峯下滑
囊炎

subluxation 半脱位

subungual haematoma
甲下血腫

supination 旋後

synchondrosis 軟骨聯合／軟骨
結合

syndactyly 併指 (趾) 畸形

syndrome, cauda equina 馬尾
症候群／馬尾綜合症

syndrome, compartment 骨筋
膜室綜合症／筋膜間隔綜合症
／腔隙綜合症

synovectomy 滑膜切除術

synovial cyst 滑膜囊腫

synovitis 滑膜炎

talipes 畸形足

talipes calcaneus 仰趾足

talipes equinovarus
馬蹄內翻足

talipes equinus 馬蹄足

talipes valgus 外翻足

talipes varus 內翻足

tendinitis 腱炎

tendo-achilles 跟腱

tendon 腱

tendon sheath 腱鞘

tenosynovitis 腱鞘滑膜炎

tetanus 破傷風

thigh 股，大腿

thumb 拇指

tissue 組織

tophus 痛風石／痛風結節／結
節腫塊

torticollis 斜頸

total elbow replacement 全肘
關節置換術

total hip replacement 全髖關
節置換術

total knee replacement 全膝關節置換術

total shoulder replacement 全肩關節置換術

traction 牽引

transplant 移植

trauma 外傷，創傷

trigger finger 板機指

ulnar neuritis 尺骨神經炎

ultrasound therapy 超音療法

union 連接

union, delayed 連接遲緩

valgus 外翻

varus 內翻

verruca vulgaris (common wart) 尋常疣

vertebra 椎骨，脊椎

vertebroplasty 椎體整形術

wart 疣

whiplash injury 類鞭梢頸傷

whitlow 化膿性指頭炎

wiring 架綫縫法 (骨折)

xanthoma 黃瘤

xenograft 異種移植物

z-plasty Z 形整形術

15 Psychiatry 精神科

abuse 濫用

abuse, alcohol 酒精濫用

abuse, drug 藥物濫用

adaptation 適應

addiction 上癮

adjustment 適應

affect 情感，情緒

affection 鍾愛

aggression 攻擊性

agoraphobia
空曠恐懼，廣場恐慌

alcoholism 酗酒

Alzheimer's disease
阿氏癡呆症

amnesia 失憶

anorexia 厭食

anorexia nervosa 神經性厭食症

antidepressant 抗抑鬱藥

antisocial personality
反社會型人格 (異常)

anxiety 焦慮

aphrodisiac 催情藥

assessment 評量，評估

assessment, clinical 臨床評量

association 聯想

attention deficit disorder
注意力缺失症
(與過份活躍症類同)

autism 自閉

behaviour 行為

behaviour, aggressive
攻擊行為

behaviour, ambivalent
矛盾情緒行為

behaviour, impulsive 衝動行為

behaviour, instinctive
本能行為

biofeedback 生理回饋

bipolar affective disorder
雙極型情緒異常

bulimia 暴食

catatonic 緊張僵直

catharsis 舒洩

character 性格

compensation 補償

compensation, over 過度補償

complex, Electra 戀父病或戀父
情結

complex, inferiority 自卑感或
自卑情結

complex, Oedipus 戀母病

compulsion 強迫行為

concept 概念

conditioning 制約，慣性建立

conduct disorder 品性異常

confabulation 虛構情節

conflict 衝突，矛盾

consciousness 清醒狀態

conversion 轉化

coping skills 因應技巧，適應
態力

counter transference 反角色
轉移

day care centre 日托中心

day hospital 日間醫院

defense mechanism 防衛機制

deinstitutionalization 機構開
放化

delirium 妄言

delusion 妄想

dementia 痴呆

denial 否認

depression 抑鬱，憂鬱

depression, involutional
更年期抑鬱，更年期憂鬱

deprivation 缺失，剝奪

despair 失望

developmental disorder
發展性障礙，成長過程障礙

disorientation 定向力障礙

displacement 轉移

dream 夢

drive 動力

dyslexia 閱讀障礙

dyspareunia 性交疼痛

ego 自我

electroconvulsive therapy (ECT) 電痙攣療法

emotion 情緒

empathy 同理心

enuresis 遺尿症

enuresis, nocturnal 夜遺尿

environment 環境

epilepsy 癲癇病 (發羊吊)

equilibrium 平衡

erection 勃起 (豎起)

exhibitationism 暴露狂

extinction 消弱，消失

factitious disorder 詐病異常，詐病症

family therapy 家庭治療

fantasy 幻想

fetishism 戀物僻

fixation 固定，固著

free association 自由聯想

frigidity 性冷感

generalized anxiety disorder 泛焦慮症

gesture 舉動

grief 悲哀

group therapy 團體治療

hallucination 幻覺

heredity 遺傳

heterosexual relationship 異性戀

histrionic personality 劇化型人格 (異常)

homosexual relationship 同性戀

hypnosis 催眠術

hypnotic 安眠藥

hypochondriasis 疑病症

hysteria 歇斯底里

Id 本我，我之本

identification 認同

identity crisis 身份危機

illusion 錯覺

image 意像 (形像)

impotence 陽萎 (性無能)

impulsive 衝動

incest 亂倫

inhibition 抑制

insight 領悟

insomnia 失眠症

instability 不穩定

instinct 本能

intelligence 智力

intelligence quotient (IQ) 智力商數

intelligence test 智力測驗

interview 會談

intoxication 中毒 (醉酒)

involution 內轉

jealousy 妒忌

judgement 判斷

latent 潛伏性

learning 學習

learning disability 學習障礙

lesbian 女同性戀者

libido 慾力，性慾

lithium 鋰

malingering 裝病

mania 狂躁症

manic-depressive 躁狂抑鬱

melancholia 情緒低落，憂鬱

memory 記憶

mental illness 精神心理病

mental retardation
　智力發育遲緩 (弱智)

mental retardation, mild grade 輕度弱智

mental retardation, moderate grade 中度弱智

mental retardation, severe grade 嚴重弱智

mood 心境

motivation 動機

mourning 哀傷

narcissistic personality
　自戀型人格 (異常)

narcolepsy 嗜睡病

neurosis 神經機能病

neurotransmitter
　神經傳導物質

obsessions 強迫思想

obsessive-compulsive
　執著強迫性

organic psychosis
　有機性精神病

orientation 定向 (方向)

panic disorder 恐慌症

paranoia 猜疑被害忘想

paraphilias 性行為對象的異常

pedophiliac 戀童症

perception 知覺

personality 性格

personality, anxious 焦慮性格

personality, extroverted
　外向性格

personality, introverted
內向性格

personality, obsessional
執著性格

personality, passive aggressive
消極侵略性格

personality, paranoid
猜疑性格

persuasion 勸導

pervasive developmental
disorder 廣泛的發展障礙

perversion 變態

phobia 恐懼

placebo 假藥

post-traumatic stress disorder
重大創傷後遺症

premature ejaculation
射精過早 (早洩)

projection 投射作用

psyche 心靈

psychiatry/psychiatrist
精神科/精神科醫生

psychoanalysis 心理分析

psychology/psychologist
心理學/心理學家

psychology, clinical
臨床心理學

psychometric tests 心理測量

psychopath 心理病態

psychosis 精神症

psychosomatic 心身性

psychotherapy 心理療法

psychotherapy, group
小組心理療法

rape 強暴

rationalization 合理化

reaction formation 反向作用

reassurance 使放心，再保證

recall 回憶

reflex 反射 (作用)

regression 退化

rehabilitation 康復

reinforcement 增強

rejection 排斥，拒絕

repression 壓抑

restitution 整復，回復，再復

ritualize 儀式化

sadism 虐待狂

schizo-affective disorder
情感型精神分裂症

schizophrenia 精神分裂症

schizophrenia, catatonic
緊張性精神分裂症

schizophrenia, paranoid
猜疑妄想精神分裂症

schizophrenia, simple
單純精神分裂症

sedative 鎮靜劑

senility 衰老

sexual dysfunction 性機能失常

**sleep walking
(somnambulism)** 夢遊病

social consciousness 社會意識

social phobia 社交恐懼症

socialization 社會化

somatic 軀體

stimulant 興奮劑，刺激藥

stress 壓力

subconscious 下意識

sublimation
昇華(作用)，理想化

substitution 取代

suggestion 暗示

suicide 自殺

superego 超我

suppression 壓制

taboo 禁忌

temperament 氣質，脾氣

therapy 治療

therapy, aversion 厭惡治療

theraphy, behaviour 行為治療

therapy, convulsive 痙攣治療

**therapy, electroconvulsive
(ECT)** 電痙攣療法

therapy, occupational
職業療法

tic 抽搐

tranquillizer 鎮靜劑

tranquillizer, major
抗精神分裂病藥

tranquillizer, minor 抗焦慮藥

transference 移情作用，角色
代入

transsexualism 變性症

transvestitism 異性裝癖

unconscious 昏迷(不省人事)

unipolar affective disorder
單極型情緒病

vocation 從業

voyeurism 窺視症，偷窺症

withdrawal 脫癮(戒除)

16 Dentistry 牙齒科

abscess 膿腫

abscess, acute alveolar
急性牙槽膿腫

abutment 橋基

adenomatoid odontogenic
tumour 腺性成釉細胞瘤
(adeno-adamantoblastoma is
old terminology)

alignment 校列

alignment, functional
功能性校列

alloy 合金

alveolectomy 牙槽緣切除術

alveolus 牙槽

alveolus cleft 牙槽裂

amalgam 汞合金

ameloblastic carcinoma
釉質癌

ameloblastoma 成釉細胞瘤
(adamantinoma,
adamantoma,
adamantoblastoma are old
terminology)

amelogenesis imperfecta
釉質生長不全

anaesthesia, extraoral
口外麻醉法

anaesthesia, inferior alveolar
nerve block 下牙槽神經麻醉

anaesthesia, intraoral
口內麻醉法

anaesthesia, nerve block
神經阻斷麻醉

analyser, occlusal 分䶝器

anchorage 牙錨基

angina, Ludwig's 膿性頜下炎

angina, Vincent's
急性潰瘍齦炎

angioneurotic oedema
血管神經性水腫

ankylosis 強直

ankylosis, jaw/
temporomandibular joint
牙關節／顳下顎關節強直

anodontia 無牙 (畸形)

anodontia, partial 部分無牙

aphthae/recurrent aphthous
ulcer 復發性口腔潰瘍

apicectomy 牙根尖切除術

appliance 口腔矯正器

appliance, orthodontic
牙矯正器

approximal 鄰接

aptyalia, aptyalism 無涎

articulation
關節，排牙，接觸面咬合

articulator 架

attachment, epithelial
上皮附着

attrition 磨損

atypical facial pain
非典型顏面痛

atypical odontalgia
非典型牙痛

B.D.S. (Bachelor of Dental
Surgery) 牙科醫學士

B.D.Sc. (Bachelor of Dental
Science) 牙理科學士

baseplate 基板

bicuspid 雙尖牙

bifurcation 分歧

bisphosphonate associated
osteonecrosis 雙膦酸鹽性頜
骨壞死

bite raising 增高

breaker, stress 應力中斷器

bridge 橋

bridge, cantilever 單端固定橋

bridge, fixed 固定橋

bridge, removable 活動橋

burr 鑽

calcification 鈣化

calculus 積石，牙垢 (牙石)

canal, accessory root 副根管

canal, inferior dental 下頜管

canal, pulp 髓管

candidiasis 念珠菌症 (鵝口瘡)

capping, pulp 蓋髓術

caries 齲，蛀牙

caries, arrested 休止齲

caries, rampant 廣佈性齲

caries, recurrent 復發性齲

carver 雕刻器

casting 鑄造

cavosurface 洞面

cement 黏固粉

cementogenesis 牙骨質成長

cementoblastoma 牙骨質瘤

cementum 牙骨質

central giant cell lesions
鉅細胞瘤 (病變)

cephalometric analysis
頭測量分析

cherubism 領骨增大症

clamp 夾

clasp 卡環

cleft 裂

cleft lip 裂唇

cleft palate 腭裂

community dentistry
社會牙醫學

complete denture/full denture
全口義齒 (假牙)

composite resin 複合樹脂

condenser, amalgam
汞合金充填器

condylectomy 髁切除術

condylotomy 髁割開術

connector 連接體

contour 外形

coping 牙蓋

core, amalgam 汞合金中軸

core, cast-gold 鑄合軸

corrosion 腐蝕

craniofacial 面顱

crevice 縫

crib 槽

crossbite 反

crown 冠

crown, jacket 甲冠

crown, veneer 罩冠

curvature, gingival 齦曲線

curve, Spee's 牙列，面曲線

cusp 牙尖

cuticle, dental 牙護膜

cyst, dental 含牙囊腫

cyst, dentigerous 含牙囊腫

dam, palate post 上腭後緣障

dam, rubber 橡皮障

decalcification 脫鈣

decay 腐蝕，蛀牙

dens in dente 牙中牙

dental hygiene 牙齒衛生

dental implant 植牙

dental laboratory 牙科工場

dental papilla 牙乳頭

dental public health
牙科公共衛生

dental subspecialties 牙科專科

dental surgeon 牙科醫生

dental surgeon assistant 牙科
手術助理員

dental technician 牙科技術員

dental therapist 牙科治療員

dental denticle 小牙

denticulus 髓石

dentine, carious 齲牙質

dentinogenesis 牙質生成

dentist 牙醫

dentistry 牙科

dentistry, conservative
修補牙科

dentistry, prosthetic 義齒牙科

dentition 出牙，牙列

denture 牙托、義齒

desensitizer 脫敏藥

devitalize 去生機

diastem, diastema 間隙

die 代型

dilaceration 彎曲牙

disease, Fordyce's
黏膜皮脂腺腫大

disease, Magitot's 牙槽骨膜炎

disease, Paget's 彎形性骨炎

disease, periodontal 牙週病

disease, Vincent's
潰瘍假膜性口炎

disharmony, occlusal　失調

dislocation 脫位

disto-occlusion 遠中

dowel 樁

drill 錐

duct, nasolacrimal 鼻淚管

duct, parotid 腮腺管

duct, Stensen's 腮腺管

duct, Wharton's 頜下腺導管

edentulous 無牙

elevator 牙挺

embrasure 楔狀隙

enamel 釉質

endodontics 牙髓治療科

epithelium, reduced enamel
縮餘釉上皮

epulis 齦瘤

erosion 磨耗

eruption 長出

erythroplakia 紅斑

excavator 挖器

exodontics 拔牙學

face-bow 面弓

facing 假牙面

family dentistry 家庭牙醫學

fibroma, odontogenic
牙纖維瘤

fibrosarcoma 口內纖維肉癌

fibrous dysplasia 骨纖維性
結構不良

filler 充填劑

filling 充填填料

filling, provisional 暫充填

filling, temporary 暫充填

film, dental 牙照片

fissure 裂縫

fistula 瘻管

flange 翼

flap 瓣

flap, surgical 外科成瓣術

floss, dental 牙線

fluoride 氟

fluorosis 氟中毒

forceps 牙鉗

fossa 窩

fracture 骨折，折斷

frenulum 繫帶

frenum 繫帶

furcate 分叉

gag 張器

gangrena oris 口腔壞疽

genioplasty 頦整形術

geographic tongue 地圖舌

geriatric dentistry/
geriodontology 老年牙醫學

gingiva 牙齦

gingivectomy 齦切除術

gingivitis 牙齦炎

gingivitis, acute ulcerative
急性潰瘍齦炎

gland, salivary 涎腺

glaze 釉料，上釉

glossopharyngeal neuralgia
舌咽神經痛

gnathology 頜理學

granuloma 肉芽腫

groove 溝

guidance 導

gutta-percha 牙膠

haemorrhage, hemorrhage
出血

halitosis 口臭

handpiece 牙機嘴

hatchet 斧

headache 頭痛

headgear 頭網裝置

headrest 頭靠

healing abutment 癒合連接體

height of contour 外形高度

hernia of pulp 牙髓疝

herpes simplex 單純疱疹

hoe 鋤刮

holder, clamp 持夾器

hygienist, dental 口腔保健員

hyperplasia 增殖

hyperplastic 增殖性的

hypersensitiveness 過敏

hypertrophy 增大

hypodontia / partial anodontia 部分無牙

hypoplastic 增殖不良

impacted tooth 阻生齒

impaction 嵌塞

implantation 植入

implant fixture 牙種植體

impression 印模

incisor 門齒

index 指數

inferior alveolar nerve 下牙槽神經

inferior dental canal 下頜神經管

infiltration 浸潤

infiltration anaesthesia 浸潤麻醉

inlay 嵌體

instrument 器具

interdigitation 牙間殆

interproximal 鄰間

intrude 向內移位

invest 包埋

jaw, edentulous 無牙頜

juvenile periodontitis 青少年牙周炎

keratocystic odontogenic tumour/odontogenic keratocyst/keratocyst 牙源性角化囊腫

lamella 板

lamina dura 硬板

leukoplakia 白斑

lever 牙桿

lichen planus 扁平苔癬

ligament 牙槽韌帶

ligature 縛綫

lingual nerve 舌神經

lining 襯料

lumen 腔

mallet 鎚

malocclusion 錯位

mandible 下頜骨

mandibular condyle 下顎髁突

margin 緣

mastication 咀嚼

maxilla 上頜骨

megadont 巨牙

melanoma 黑素癌

method, cephalometric
  頭測量法

microdont 小牙

microglossia 小舌

micrognathia 小頜 (畸形)

migration, mesial 向中移位

model 模型

molar 大臼齒

mounting 裝置

mucosa 黏膜

mumps 流行性腮腺炎

necrosis, pulp 髓壞死

neuralgia dentalis 牙神經痛

neurosis 神經官能病

numbness, mouth 口麻痹

obturator 充填體

occlusion 殆咬合

odontoblast 成牙質細胞

odontoclast 破牙質細胞

odontogenic tumour
  牙源性腫瘤

onlay 嵌體

operation, flap 成瓣手術

operculum 蓋

oral 口的

oral and maxillofacial surgery
  口腔頜面外科

oral medicine 口腔內科

oral surgery 口腔外科

orthodontics 牙齒矯正科學

orthognathic 正頜的

orthognathic surgery 正頜外科

ossifying fibroma 骨化性
  纖維瘤

osseointegration 骨整合

osteitis 骨炎

osteointegrated implant
  牙床骨植根術

osteoma, dental 牙骨質瘤

osteomyelitis, alveolar
　牙槽骨髓炎

osteoradionecrosis 放射性
　骨壞死

overdenture 覆蓋義齒

overbite 覆

pack 塞填

paediatric dentistry 兒童齒科

paedodontics 小兒齒科

palatal 腭的

palsy, Bell's (facial paralysis)
　面神經麻痺

papilla 牙乳頭

partial denture 局部義齒
　（假牙）

pattern, wax 蠟型

pearl, enamel 釉珠

pemphigoid 類天疱瘡

pemphigus 天疱瘡

periapical 根尖周的

pericoronitis 冠周炎

periodontics 牙周學

periodontology 牙週治療科

periostitis 骨膜炎

pharynx, oral 口咽

plaque 斑，菌膜

pleomorphic adenoma
　多形性腺瘤

pocket 袋

polymer 聚合體

polyp 息肉

pontic 橋體，假牙

porcelain 瓷

post 牙樁

premolar 前磨牙

preparation, cavity 製洞

probe 牙周探針

prognathism 凸頜畸形

prophylaxis 預防

prosthesis, dental 義齒

prosthetics 義齒科

prosthodontics 修復齒科

protrusion 前突

proximo- 鄰

ptyalism 流涎過多

pulpcap 蓋髓劑

pulpectomy 牙髓切除術

pulpitis 牙髓炎

pulpotomy 牙髓切斷術

radiolucency 射線透射

radio-opaque 射線阻射

ranula 舌下囊腫

reamer 擴孔鑽

reattachment 再附著

rebasing 墊底術

recession 退縮

record 牙科記錄

reflex 反射 (作用)

registration, occlusal 𬌗架記錄

rehabilitation, oral
口腔機能恢復

relapse 復發

relining 重襯

replantation 再植

resorption 吸回

rest 支托

restoration 修復

retrude 後移

ridge 脊

roentgenogram, dental
口腔造影

saddle 鞍基

saliva 涎

scaler 刮器

screw, anchor 錨凹螺絲

sensitivity, tooth surface
牙面敏感度

separator 分牙器

septum 中隔

shade-guide 色標

shoulder 肩

sialogram 涎管照相造影

sialolithiasis 涎石成形病

silicate 矽酸鹽

sinusitis, maxillary 上頜竇炎

socket 槽

solder 銲

spatula 調刀

splint, dental 牙夾

squamous cell carcinoma
鱗狀細胞癌

stomatitis 口炎

strip 磨帶，帶

suction 抽吸

sulcus 溝

supernumerary tooth 多生齒

support 支持

surveyor 測量器

syringe, jet 噴射器

teething 出牙

temporomandibular 顳下頜的

temporomandibular joint
dislocation 下頜關節脫位

temporomandibular joint pain dysfunction
顳下頜關節紊亂綜合症

test, pulp 髓試法

tester, pulp 試髓器

tetracycline stain 四環素牙斑

titanium bone plate 鈦骨板

titanium dental implant
鈦牙種植體

tongue-tie 舌結

tooth-shade 牙色

torch 吹熠器

torus 隆凸

traction 牽引

tray 托盤

trigeminal neuralgia
三义神經痛

trimmer 修整器

trismus 牙關緊閉

tubercle 結節

tumour 腫瘤 (癌)

ulcer 潰瘍

varnish 塗劑

verrucous carcinoma 疣狀癌

vibrator 顫動器

vitality 生機

wear 戴，磨損

wedge 楔

wheel 輪

xerostomia 缺涎病

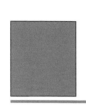

Appendix I
附錄一

A. Anaesthesia 麻醉科

acidosis 酸中毒

alkalosis 鹼中毒

amnesia 失憶，失憶病

anaesthesia, anesthesia
麻醉，麻醉科

anaesthesia, caudal 脊尾麻醉

anaesthesia, epidural
硬膜外麻醉

anaesthesia, general 全身麻醉

anaesthesia, local 局部麻醉

anaesthesia, regional 部位麻醉

anaesthesia, spinal 脊柱麻醉

anaesthesiology/
anaesthesiologist
麻醉科/麻醉科醫生

anaesthetic gases 麻醉氣體

anaesthestist 麻醉科醫生

analgesia 痛覺缺乏

arterial blood gas 動脈血氣壓

carbon dioxide 二氧化碳

central venous pressure
中樞靜脈(血)壓

cyanosis 發紫，發紺

endotracheal intubation
氣管內插管法

endotracheal tube 氣管內管

euphoria 飄飄欲仙

hypertension 高血壓

hyperventilate 呼吸過度

hypotension 低血壓

hypothermia 低溫

hypoxia 缺氧

induction 麻醉引發

intravenous infusion 靜脈輸注

intravenous injection 靜脈注射

mask 面罩

monitor 監察

muscle relaxant 肌弛藥

narcotic 麻醉藥

nitrous oxide 一氧化氮

oxygen 氧

paralysis 癱瘓 (麻痺)

reversal 逆轉

ventilate 呼吸，換氣

ventilation, artificial 人工呼吸

ventilation, manual 人力呼吸

ventilation, mechanical
機械呼吸

ventilator 呼吸機

B. Community Medicine 社會醫學

accuracy 準確性

analysis 分析

analysis, qualitative 定性分析

analysis, quantitative 定量分析

coefficient 係數

cohort analysis 斷代分析

computer analysis 電腦分析

contact 接觸

correlation 相關，聯繫

correlation coefficient
相關係數

epidemic 病疫

epidemiology 分佈病學

industrial health 工業衛生

insect vector 昆蟲媒介

isolation 隔離

morbidity rate 發病率

mortality rate 死亡率

mortality rate, infant
  嬰兒死亡率 (一歲以下)

mortality rate, maternal
  孕婦死亡率

mortality rate, neonatal
  新生期嬰兒死亡率
  (一月以下)

mortality rate, perinatal
  產期嬰兒死亡率 (一週以下)

normal distribution 常態分析

normal probability curve
  常態概率曲線

prevalence rate 流行率

probability 或然率

quarantine
  檢疫，檢疫期，檢疫所

quotient 商數

rate 率

ratio 比率

sampling 抽樣

sampling, random 隨機抽樣

sensitivity 敏性

significance 顯著

significant difference
  顯著性差異

specificity 特性

standard deviation 標準偏差

standard error 標準差誤

statistical analysis 統計分析

statistics 統計學

surveillance 監視

variable 變數

World Health Organization
  (WHO) 世界衛生組織

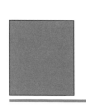

Appendix II
附錄二

A. Artery and Vein 動靜脈

acetabular a. & v. 髖臼動靜脈

alveolar, inferior, a. & v.
下牙槽動靜脈

alveolar, superior, a. & v.
上牙槽動靜脈

angular a. & v. 內　動靜脈

aorta 主動脈

appendicular a. & v.
闌尾動靜脈

arcuate a. & v. 弓形動靜脈

auricular, posterior, a. & v.
耳後動靜脈

axillary a. & v. 腋動靜脈

azygos vein 奇靜脈

brachial a. & v. 臂動靜脈

brachiocephalic a.
(innominate) 頭臂動脈

buccal a. & v. 頰動靜脈

bulbourethral a. & v.
尿道球動靜脈

caecal (cecal) a. & v.
盲腸動靜脈

carotid, common, artery
頸總動脈

carotid, external, artery
頸外動脈

carotid, internal, artery
頸內動脈

cerebellar, inferior anterior, a.
& v. 小腦下前動靜脈

cerebellar, inferior posterior,
a. & v. 小腦下後動靜脈

cerebellar, superior, a. & v.
小腦上動靜脈

cerebral, anterior, a. & v.
大腦前動靜脈

cerebral, middle, a. & v.
大腦中動靜脈

cerebral, posterior, a. & v.
大腦後動靜脈

cervical, ascending, a. & v.
頸升動靜脈

cervical, profunda, a. & v.
頸深動靜脈

choroidal a. & v. 脈絡膜動靜脈

ciliary, anterior, a. & v.
狀前動靜脈

ciliary, posterior, a. & v.
狀後動靜脈

circumflex femoral a. & v.
旋股動靜脈

circumflex humeral a. & v.
旋肱動靜脈

circumflex iliac a. & v.
旋髂動靜脈

circumflex scapular a. & v.
旋骨胛動靜脈

coeliac a. & v. (celiac)
腹腔動靜脈

colic, left, a. & v. 結腸左動靜脈

colic, middle, a. & v.
結腸中動靜脈

colic, right, a. & v.
結腸右動靜脈

communicating, anterior,
a. & v. 前交通動靜脈

communicating, posterior,
a. & v. 後交通動靜脈

coronary, left, a. & v.
左冠狀動靜脈

coronary, right, a. & v.
右冠狀動靜脈

dental a. & v. 牙髓動靜脈

digital, dorsal, a. & v.
指 (趾) 背動靜脈

digital, palmar, a. & v.
指掌側動靜脈

dorsalis nasi a. & v.
鼻梁動靜脈

dorsalis pedis a. & v.
足背動靜脈

dorsalis penis a. & v.
陰莖動靜脈

epigastric, inferior, a. & v.
腹壁下動靜脈

epigastric, superficial, a. & v.
腹壁淺動靜脈

epigastric, superior, a. & v.
腹壁上動靜脈

ethmoidal, anterior, a. & v.
篩前動靜脈

ethmoidal, posterior, a. & v.
篩後動靜脈

facial, a. & v. 面動靜脈

femoral v. 股內靜脈

femoral, profunda, a. & v.
股深動靜脈

femoral, superficial, a. & v.
股淺動靜脈

fibular, a. & v. 腓動靜脈

gastric, left, a. & v.
胃左動靜脈

gastric, right, a. & v.
胃右動靜脈

gastric, short, a. & v.
胃短動靜脈

gastroduodenal a. & v.
胃十二指腸動靜脈

gastroepiploic, left, a. & v.
胃網膜左動靜脈

gastroepiploic, right, a. & v.
胃網膜右動靜脈

genicular, inferior, a. & v.
膝下動靜脈

genicular, middle, a. & v.
膝中動靜脈

genicular, superior, a. & v.
膝上動靜脈

gluteal, inferior, a. & v.
臀下動靜脈

gluteal, superior, a. & v.
臀上動靜脈

haemorrhoidal, inferior, a. & v.
直腸下動靜脈

haemorrhoidal, middle, a. & v.
直腸中動靜脈

haemorrboidal, superior,
a. & v. 直腸上動靜脈

hemiazygos vein 半奇靜脈

hepatic, common, a. & v.
肝總動靜脈

hepatic, left, a. & v. 肝左動靜脈

hepatic, proper, artery
肝固有動脈

hepatic, right, a. & v.
肝右動靜脈

ileal a. & v. 回腸動靜脈

ileocaecal a. & v. 回結腸動靜脈

iliac, common, a. & v.
髂總動靜脈

iliac, external, a. & v.
髂外動靜脈

iliac, internal, a. & v.
髂內動靜脈

iliolumbar a. & v. 髂腰動靜脈

infraorbital a. & v. 眶下動靜脈

intercostal a. & v. 肋間動靜脈

interosseous a. & v. 骨間動靜脈

jugular vein, external 頸外靜脈

jugular vein, internal 頸內靜脈

labial a. & v. 陰唇動靜脈

lacrimal a. & v. 激腺動靜脈

laryngeal a. & v. 喉動靜脈

lingual a. & v. 舌動靜脈

malleolar, lateral, a. & v.
外踝動靜脈

malleolar, medial, a. & v.
內踝動靜脈

mammary, internal, a. & v.
胸廓內動靜脈

masseteric a. & v. 咬肌動靜脈

maxillary a. & v. 上頜動靜脈

meningeal a. & v. 腦膜動靜脈

mesenteric, inferior, a. & v.
腸系膜下動靜脈

mesenteric, superior, a. & v.
腸系膜上動靜脈

metacarpal a. & v. 掌動靜脈

metatarsal a. & v. 跖動靜脈

nutrient a. & v. 滋養動靜脈

obturator a. & v. 閉孔動靜脈

occipital a. & v. 枕動靜脈

ophthalmic a. & v. 眼動靜脈

ovarian a. & v. 卵巢動靜脈

palatine a. & v. 腭動靜脈

pancreaticoduodenal, inferior
胰十二指腸下動靜脈

pancreaticoduodenal, superior
胰十二指腸上動靜脈

penis a. & v. 陰莖動靜脈

perineal a. & v. 會陰動靜脈

peroneal a. & v. 腓動靜脈

phrenic inferior a. & v.
膈下動靜脈

phrenic superior a. & v.
膈上動靜脈

plantar a. & v. 足底動靜脈

popliteal a. & v. 膕動靜脈

portal v. 門靜脈

pudental a. & v. 陰部動靜脈

pulmonary, left, a. & v.
肺左動靜脈

pulmonary, right, a. & v.
肺右動靜脈

radial a. & v. 橈動靜脈

radial collateral a. & v.
橈側副動靜脈

renal a. & v. 腎動靜脈

retinal a. & v. 視網膜動靜脈

sacral a. & v. 骶動靜脈

saphenous vein, long 大隱靜脈

saphenous vein, short
　小隱靜脈

sigmoid a. & v.
　乙狀結腸動靜脈

spermatic a. & v. 精索動靜脈

spinal, anterior, a. & v.
　脊髓前動靜脈

spinal, posterior, a. & v.
　脊髓後動靜脈

subclavian a. & v.
　鎖骨下動靜脈

subcostal a. & v. 肋下動靜脈

sublingual a. & v. 舌下動靜脈

subscapular a. & v.
　肩胛下動靜脈

supraorbital a. & v.
　眶上動靜脈

suprarenal a. & v.
　腎上腺動靜脈

tarsal a. & v. 跗動靜脈

temporal a. & v. 顳動靜脈

testicular a. & v. 睪丸動靜脈

thoracic a. & v. 胸動靜脈

thoracoacromial a. & v.
　胸肩峰動靜脈

thoracodorsal a. & v.
　胸背動靜脈

thyroid, inferior, a. & v.
　甲狀腺下動靜脈

thyroid, superior, a. & v.
　甲狀腺上動靜脈

tibial, anterior, a. & v.
　脛前動靜脈

tibial, posterior, a. & v.
　脛後動靜脈

tympanic a. & v. 鼓室動靜脈

ulnar a. & v. 尺動靜脈

ulnar collateral a. & v.
　尺側副動靜脈

umbilical a. & v. 臍動靜脈

uterine a. & v. 子宮動靜脈

vaginal a. & v. 陰道動靜脈

vena cava, inferior 下腔靜脈

vena cava, superior 上腔靜脈

vertebral a. & v. 椎動靜脈

vesical a. & v. 膀胱動靜脈

B. Nerves 神經

abducent nerve 外展神經

accessory nerve 副神經

alveolar nerve inferior
  下頜牙槽神經

alveolar nerve superior
  上頜牙槽神經

anococcygeal nerve 肛尾神經

auricular nerve, posterior
  耳後神經

auriculotemporal nerve
  耳顳神經

axillary nerve 腋神經

cervical nerve 頸神經

ciliary nerve 睫狀神經

cochlear nerve 聽覺神經

cutaneous nerve 皮神經

digital nerve 指 (趾) 神經

dorsal nerve of clitoris
  陰蒂背神經

dorsal nerve of penis
  陰莖背神經

facial nerve 面神經

femoral nerve 股神經

frontal nerve 額神經

genitofemoral nerve
  生殖股神經

glossopharyngeal nerve
  舌咽神經

gluteal nerve inferior 臀下神經

gluteal nerve superior
  臀上神經

hypoglossal nerve 舌下神經

intercostal nerve 肋間神經

infraorbital nerve 眶下神經

laryngeal nerve recurrent
  喉返神經

laryngeal nerve superior
  喉上神經

lingual nerve 舌神經

long thoracic nerve 胸長神經

lumbar nerve 腰神經

mandibular nerve 下頜神經

maxillary nerve 上頜神經

mental nerve 頦神經

musculocutaneous nerve
  肌皮神經

obturator nerve 閉孔神經

oculomotor nerve 動眼神經

olfactory nerve 嗅神經

ophthalmic nerve 眼神經

optic nerve 視神經

palatine nerve 腭神經

perineal nerve 會陰神經

phrenic nerve 膈神經

pudendal nerve 陰部神經

radial nerve 橈神經

sacral nerve 骶神經

saphenous nerve 隱神經

stapedial nerve 鐙骨神經

subcostal nerve 肋下神經

supraclavicular nerve
鎖骨上神經

sural nerve 腓腸神經

thoracodorsal nerve 胸背神經

tibial nerve 脛神經

trigeminal nerve 三叉神經

trochlear nerve 滑輪神經

ulnar nerve 尺神經

vagal nerve 迷走神經

C. Bones 骨骼

acetabulum 髖臼骨

atlas 寰椎

axis 軸椎

basilar 底骨

calcaneus 跟骨

capitate 頭狀骨

carpal 腕骨

clavicle 鎖骨

coccyx 尾骨

cuboid 骰骨

cuneiform of hand 三角骨

cuneiform of foot 楔骨

ethmoid 篩骨

femur 股骨

fibula 腓骨

frontal 額骨

hamate 鉤骨

humerus 肱骨

hyoid 舌骨

ilium 髂骨

ischium 坐骨

lunate 半月骨

mandible 下頜骨

mastoid 乳突狀骨

maxilla 上頜骨

metacarpal 掌骨

metatarsal 蹠骨

nasal 鼻骨

navicular 舟骨

occipital 枕骨

orbiculare 環狀骨

palatine 腭骨

parietal 頂骨

patella 膝蓋骨

phalange 指(趾)骨

pisiform 碗豆骨

pterygoid 翼狀骨

pubis 恥骨

radius 橈骨

rib 肋骨

sacrum 骶骨

scaphoid 舟狀骨

scapula 肩胛骨

sesamoid 種子狀骨

sphenoid 蝶骨

sternum 胸骨

talus 距骨

tarsal 跗骨

temporal 顳骨

tibia 脛骨

trapezium 斜方骨

trapezoid 稜形骨

triquetrum 楔骨

ulna 尺骨

vertebra 椎骨

zygoma 顴骨

D. Joints 關節

acromio-clavicular
  肩峰鎖骨關節
ankle 踝關節
atlanto-axial 寰軸關節
atlanto-occipital 寰枕關節

calcaneo-cuboid 跟骰關節
carpal 腕關節
carpometacarpal 腕掌關節
costochondral 肋軟骨關節
costovertebral 肋椎關節

elbow 肘關節

hip 髖關節

interphalangeal 指 (趾)
  骨間關節

knee 膝關節

metacarpophalangeal
  掌指關節

midcarpal 腕中關節
midtarsal 跗中關節

patellofemoral 髕股關節

radio-ulnar 橈尺關節

sacrococcygeal 骶尾關節
sacro-iliac 骶髂關節
shoulder 肩關節
sternoclavicular 胸鎖關節
sternocostal 胸肋關節
subtalar
  距跟關節 (踝骨下關節)

talocalcanean 距跟關節
talonavicular 距舟關節
tarsometatarsal 跗蹠關節
tibiofibular 脛腓關節

wrist 腕關節

E. Muscles 肌

abductor digiti minimi
小指展肌

abductor hallucis　　展肌

abductor pollicis brevis
拇短展肌

abductor pollicis longus
拇長展肌

adductor brevis 短收肌

adductor hallucis　　收肌

adductor longus 長收肌

adductor magnus 大收肌

adductor minimus 小收肌

adductor pollicis 拇收肌

anconeus 肘(後)肌

antitragicus 對耳屏肌

articularis genu 膝關節肌

aryepiglotticus 杓會壓肌

biceps brachii 肱二頭肌

biceps femoris 股二頭肌

brachialis 肱肌

brachioradialis 肱橈肌

buccinator 頰肌

buccopharyngeus 頰咽肌

bulbocavernosus 球海綿體肌

bulbospongiosus 球海綿體肌

ciliary 睫狀肌

coccygeus 尾骨肌

coracobrachialis 喙肱肌

cremaster 睪提肌

cricopharyngeus 環咽肌

deltoid 三角肌

depressor labii inferioris
下唇方肌

detrusor, urinary 逼尿肌

digastric 二腹肌

dilator, pupil 瞳孔開大肌

erector, spine 骶棘肌

extensor carpi radialis brevis
橈側腕短伸肌

extensor carpi radialis longus
橈側腕長伸肌

extensor carpi ulnaris
尺側腕伸肌

extensor digitorum 指總伸肌

extensor digitorum brevis
趾短伸肌

extensor digitorum longus
趾長伸肌

extensor hallucis brevis
短伸肌

extensor hallucis longus
長伸肌

extensor indicis 食指伸肌

extensor pollicis brevis
拇短伸肌

extensor pollicis longus
拇長伸肌

flexor carpi radialis
橈側腕屈肌

flexor carpi ulnaris
尺側腕屈肌

flexor digiti minimi brevis
小指短屈肌

flexor digitorum brevis
趾短屈肌

flexor digitorum longus
趾長屈肌

flexor digitorum profundus
指深屈肌

flexor digitorum sublimis
指淺屈肌

flexor hallucis brevis   短屈肌

flexor hallucis longus
    長屈肌

flexor pollicis brevis 拇短屈肌

flexor pollicis longus 拇長屈肌

frontalis, venter 額肌

gastrocnemius 腓腸肌

genioglossus 頦舌肌

glossopharyngeus 舌咽肌

gluteus maximus 臀小肌

gluteus medius 臀大肌

gluteus minimus 臀中肌

gracilis 股薄肌

hyoglossus 舌骨舌肌

iliacus 髂肌

iliococcygeus 髂尾肌

iliopsoas 髂腰肌

interossei, dorsal 骨間背側肌

interossei, palmar 骨間掌側肌

interossei, plantar 骨間跖側

ischiocavernosus 坐骨海綿體肌

latissimus dorsi 背闊肌

levator ani 肛提肌

levator labii, inferior 下唇提肌

levator labii, superior
    上唇方肌

levator palpebrae superioris
    上瞼提肌

levator scapulae 肩胛提肌

levator veli palatini 腭帆提肌

masseter 咬肌

mentalis 頦肌

mylohyoideus 下頜舌骨肌

nasolabialis 鼻唇肌

obliquus externus abdominis
  腹外斜肌
obliquus internus abdominis
  腹內斜肌
obturator externus 閉孔外肌
obturator internus 閉孔內肌
omohyoideus 肩胛舌骨肌
orbicularis oculi 眼幹匝肌
orbicularis oris 口幹匝肌

palmaris brevis 掌短肌
palmaris longus 掌長肌
pectineus 恥骨肌
pectoralis major 胸大肌
pectoralis minor 胸小肌
perinei 會陰肌
piriformis 梨狀肌
plantaris 跖肌
platysma 頸闊肌
popliteus 膕肌
pronator quadratus 旋前方肌
pronator teres 旋前圓肌

psoas major 腰大肌
psoas minor 腰小肌
pterygoid, lateral 翼外肌
pterygoid, medial 翼內肌
puborectalis 恥骨直腸肌
pubovaginalis 恥骨陰道肌
pubovesicalis 恥骨膀胱肌
pyramidalis 錐狀肌

quadratus lumborum 腰方肌
quadriceps femoris 股四頭肌

rectococcygeus 直腸尾骨肌
recto-urethralis 直腸尿道肌
recto-uterinus 直腸子宮肌
rectovesicalis 直腸膀胱肌
rectus abdominis 腹直肌
rectus femoris 股直肌
rhomboid major 大菱形肌
rhomboid minor 小菱形肌

sacrospinalis 骶棘肌
sartorius 縫匠肌
scalenus anterior 前斜角肌
scalenus medius 中斜角肌
scalenus posterior 後斜角肌

semimembranosus 半膜肌

semitendinosus 半腱肌

serratus anterior 前鋸肌

serratus posterior 後鋸肌

soleus 比目魚肌

sphincter 括約肌

sphincter ani externus
　肛門外括約肌

sphincter ani internus
　肛門內括約肌

sphincter urethrae
　尿道膜部括約肌

sphincter vesicae 膀胱括約肌

spinalis 棘肌

sternocleidomastoid
　胸鎖乳突肌

sternohyoid 胸骨舌骨肌

sternothyroid 胸骨甲狀肌

styloglossus 莖突舌肌

stylohyoideus 莖突舌骨肌

stylopharyngeus 莖突咽肌

subclavius 鎖骨下肌

subscapularis 肩胛下肌

supinator 旋後肌

supraspinatus 岡上肌

temporalis 顳肌

tensor tympani 鼓膜張肌

tensor veli palatini 腭帆張肌

teres major 大圓肌

teres minor 小圓肌

tibialis anterior 脛骨前肌

tibialis posterior 脛骨後肌

tragicus 耳屏肌

transversospinalis 棘橫肌

transversus abdominis 腹橫肌

transversus perinei profundus
　會陰深橫肌

transversus perinei
　superficialis 會陰淺橫肌

trapezius 斜方肌

triceps brachii 肱三頭肌

uvula 懸壅垂肌

vastus intermedius 股間肌

vastus lateralis 股外肌

vastus medialis 股內肌

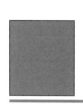

Appendix III
附錄三

A. Laboratory Tests 化驗

1. Complete blood count (CBC) 血細胞數量檢查

basophil 嗜鹼白血細胞

blood smear 血液塗片

differential count
白血細胞分類計數

eosinophil 嗜伊紅白血細胞

erythrocyte sedimentation rate (ESR) 血球沉降率

haematocrit, hematocrit
紅血細胞壓積量

haemoglobin (Hgb), hemoglobin 血紅素

lymphocyte 淋巴細胞

monocyte 單核白血細胞

neutrophil (polymorphonuclear PMN)
中性多核白血細胞

platelet 血小板

red blood cell (RBC)
紅血細胞 (紅血球)

reticulocyte 網狀紅血細胞

white blood cell (WBC)
白血細胞 (白血球)

2. Liver function tests (LFT)
肝功能化驗

albumin 清蛋白

alkaline phosphatase
鹼性磷酸酶

bilirubin 膽紅質
  direct (conjugated)
  直接膽紅質 (結合後)
  indirect (unconjugated)
  間接膽紅質 (未結合)

globulin 球蛋白

lactate dehydrogenase (LDH)
乳酸脫氫酶

serum glutamic-oxalacetic
  transaminase(SGOT)
  谷草轉氨酶
serum glutamic-pyruvic
  transaminase (SGPT)
  谷丙轉氨酶

total protein 蛋白總量

3. Rental function tests
腎功能化驗

bicarbonate (HCO₃) 碳酸氫鹽
blood urea nitrogen (BUN)
  血尿素氮

chloride (Cl) 氯

creatinine 肌酸

creatinine clearance
  肌酸　消除率

potassium (K) 鉀

sodium (Na) 鈉

urea 尿素

4. Other blood tests
其他血液化驗

α feto protein 甲類胎蛋白

amylase 澱粉酶

blood culture
  血中細菌培殖

calcium (Ca) 鈣

carcino-embryonic antigen
(CEA) 癌胚抗原

cholesterol 膽固醇

creatinine phosphokinase
(CPK) 肌酐磷酸激酶

glucose 葡萄糖
  fasting glucose 禁食後血糖量
  random glucose 隨機血糖量
  tolerance test 糖耐量

hepatitis A antigen
  甲類肝炎抗原

iron 鐵量
  total iron binding capacity
  (TIBC) 鐵結合能量

lactic acid 乳酸

lipase 脂酶

lipids, total 總脂肪

lipoprotein electrophoresis
  電泳脂肪蛋白分離

magnesium 鎂

osmolality 滲透性

phosphatase, acid 酸性磷酸酶

phosphatase, alkaline
  鹼性磷酸酶

phosphate 磷酸

phospholipid 磷脂

protein electrophoresis
  電泳蛋白分離

triglyceride 三酸甘油脂

uric acid 尿酸

VDRL 梅毒化驗

5. *Urinalysis* 尿化驗

acetone 丙酮

albumin 清蛋白

bilirubin 膽紅質

calcium 鈣

cast 管型
  granular 顆粒
  hyaline 透明

catecholamine 兒茶酚胺

chorionic gonadotrophin
  絨毛膜促性腺激素

colour 顏色

crystal 結晶

culture and sensitivit
細菌培殖與感應化驗

cytology （癌）細胞

diastase 澱粉酶

epithelial cells 上皮細胞

glucose 葡萄糖

ketone 酮

microscopy 顯微檢驗

pH 酸鹼度

pus 膿

red blood cell (RBC)
紅血細胞（紅血球）

specific gravity 比重

urobilin 尿膽質

urobilinogen 尿膽質元

white blood cell (WBC)
白血細胞（白血球）

6. *Arterial blood gas*
動脈血氣壓化驗

CO_2 content 二氧化碳含量

pCO_2 二氧化碳壓

pH 酸鹼度

pO_2 氧氣壓

7. *Clotting studies*
凝血化驗

bleeding time 流血時間

clotting time 凝血時間

fibrinogen 纖維蛋白

fibrinogen degradation
product 纖維蛋白分解產物

partial thromboplastin time
部分凝血質時間

prothrombin time
凝血酵素原時間

8. *Cerebrospinal fluid (CSF)*
脊髓液化驗

blood cell 血細胞

culture and sensitivity
　細菌培殖與感應化驗
glucose 糖

protein 蛋白質

9. Sputum analysis
　痰化驗
acid fast bacillus (AFB)
　抗酸桿菌

culture and sensitivity
　細菌培殖與感應化驗

cytology (癌) 細胞

smear 塗片

10. Stool analysis 糞化驗
fat 脂肪

occult blood 潛血
ova and parasite 寄生蟲與卵

11. Other tests 其他檢驗
basal metabolic rate (BMR)
　基本新陳代謝率

cardiac output 心輸出量
central venous pressure
　中樞靜脈壓

electrocardiogram (ECG)
　心電圖
electroencephalogram (EEG)
　腦電圖
electromyogram (EMG)
　肌電圖

pulmonary artery wedge
　pressure 肺動脈嵌壓

B. Special Investigations 特別檢驗

amniocentesis 胎膜穿刺

biopsy 活組織檢驗
blood culture 血中細菌培殖

bone marrow 骨髓化驗
bronchoscopy 支氣管鏡檢查

colonoscopy 結腸鏡檢查

cystoscopy 膀胱鏡檢查

cystometrogram
　膀胱內壓描記檢查

digital subtraction
　angiography (DSA)
　電腦數碼相減血管造影

endoscopic retrograde
　cholangiopancreatography
　(ERCP) 內窺鏡肝胰管造影

endoscopy 內窺鏡檢查

lumbar puncture 腰椎穿刺

magnetic resonance imaging
　(MRI) 磁力共振造影

pericardiocentesis 心包膜穿刺

pericentesis 腹膜穿刺

peritoneal lavage 腹腔灌洗

proctoscopy 肛門鏡檢查

sigmoidoscopy 乙狀結腸鏡

thoracocentesis 胸腹穿刺

upper endoscopy 腸胃鏡檢查

ventricular tapping 腦室穿刺

C. Radiological Tests 放射檢驗

angiogram/arteriogram
　動脈造影

barium enema 鋇灌腸造影

barium follow through
　鋇餐隨入小腸造影

barium meal 鋇餐造影

barium swallow 鋇吞咽造影

cholangiogram, intravenous
　靜脈注射膽管造影

cholecystogram, oral 膽囊造影

computerized tomography
　(CT) 電腦切片掃描

cystogram 膀胱造影

lymphangiography 淋巴管造影

magnetic resonance imaging
(MRI) 磁力共振造影

myelogram 脊髓造影

plain X-ray 平片造影

positron emission tomograph
(PET) 正電子掃描

sinogram 竇管造影

tomography 切層造影

ultrasound scan,
ultrasonography
超聲波掃描

urethrogram 尿道造影

urogram, antegrade
順行注射泌尿系統造影

urogram, intravenous
靜脈注射泌尿系統造影

urogram, retrograde
逆行注射泌尿系統造影

venogram 靜脈造影

X-ray abdomen 腹部平片造影

X-ray chest 胸部平片造影

X-ray skull 頭顱平片造影

Radioactive scans
放射元素掃描

bone scan 骨骼放射掃描

brain scan 放射性腦掃描

renal scan 放射性腎掃描

skeletal scan
全身骨骼放射掃描

thyroid scan 甲狀腺放射掃描

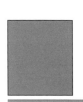

Appendix IV
附錄四

Instruments 儀器

catheter 導管
curette 刮器

diathermy 透熱燒灼機
dilator 擴張器

forceps 鉗

haemostat 止血鉗

needle 針

needle holder 針持

periosteal elevator 骨膜刮
probe 探針

scalpel 解剖刀
suction 抽吸
suture 縫術，縫綫
suture, absorbable 吸收性縫綫
suture, non-absorbable
　不吸收性縫綫
syringe 注射器 (針筒)

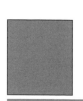

Appendix V
附錄五

A. Abbreviations 縮寫

a.c.	**ante cibum** 飯前
a.p.	**ante prandium** 飯前
b.i.d.	**bis in die** 每日二次
c̄	**cum** 和，與
caps.	**capsula** 膠囊
c.c.	**cubic centimetre** 立方厘米
gtt, gutt	**gutta** 滴
i.m.	**intramuscular** 肌內
i.s.q.	**in status quo** 維持原狀
i.v.	**intravenous** 靜脈內
p.c.	**post cibum** 飯後
p.m.	**post mortem** 驗屍
p.p.	**post prandial** 飯後

p.r.n.	**pro re nata** 需要時
Px	**recipe** 處方
q.alt.h.	**quaque alterna hora** 每隔一小時
q.d.	**quaque die** 每日
q.h.	**quaque hora** 每小時
q.i.d.	**quattuor in die** 每日四次
q.u.s.	**quantum ue satis** 數量不足
sig.	**signa** 用法
stat	**statim** 立即
suppos	**suppositorium** 塞肛
syr	**syrup** 糖水
tab	**tabella** 丸
t.i.d.	**ter in die** 每日三次
us.ext.	**usus externa** 外用
us.int.	**usus interna** 內服

B. Prefixes/Suffixes 前綴與後綴

		Example
a-, an-	無，缺	**analgesia, aseptic**
adeno-	腺	**adenoma**
-algia	痛	**myalgia**
angio-	血管	**angiogram**
ante-	前	**antenatal**
anti-	抗	**antibiotic**
aqua-, aqui-	水	**aqueous humour**
arteri-	動脈	**arteriosclerosis**

arthr-	關節	**arthritis**
auto-	自身	**auto-immune**
bi-	雙	**bicuspid**
bili-	膽汁	**bilirubin**
bio-	生命	**biopsy**
blasto-, blast-	胚	**neuroblastoma**
brachy-	短	**brachydactyly**
brady-	遲緩	**bradycardia**
bronchi-, broncho-	支氣管	**bronchitis**
calci-	石灰，鈣	**calcificatioin**
card-, cardi-, cardio-	心	**carditis**
-cardia	心	**brachycardia**
-cele	腫	**cystocele**
-centesis	穿刺	**pericentesis**
centi-	百	**centimetre**
chol-, chole-, cholo-	膽	**cholecystitis**
cholangio-	膽管	**cholangitis**
chondr-, chondro-	輭骨	**chondroma**
-cide	殺	**bacteriocidal**
co-	聯合	**cooperate**
contra-	反對	**contraception**
cysti-, cysto	膀胱，囊	**cystocele**
dent-, denti-, dens-	牙	**dentition**
des-, dis-,	分解，去，脫	**desensitize**
dextro-	右	**dextrocardia**
dia-	透	**diathermy**

		Example
dis-	分離	disconnect
-duction	導	conduction
dys-	不良，困難	dysuria
-ectasis	擴張	telangiectasis
-ectomy	割除術	splenectomy
electro-	電子	electrophoresis
-emia	血	anaemia
end-, endo-	內	endocarditis
enter-, entero-	腸	enteritis
epi-	上，表面	epiglottis
equi-	平等	equivalence
eu-	好	euthyroid
ex-	外，出	excoriation
extra-	外	extravasation
-form	形，樣	pisiform
gastr-, gastro	胃	gastroscopy
-genesis	產生	glucogenesis
-glossia	舌	macroglossia
-gram	圖，造影	angiogram
-graph	記錄	photograph
gyn-, gynae-, gynaeco-	女性	gynaecology
haem-, haemato-, haemo-	血	haemostasis
hemi-	半	hemostasis
hepat-, hepatico-, hepato-,	肝	hemiplegia
hydro-	水	hepatitis

		Example
hyp-, hypo-,	下	hydronephrosis
hyper-	過多，超過	hypochondrium
-iasis, -asis	病	hyperaemia
iatro-	醫藥	urolithiasis
-ible	可能，易於	iatrogenic
im-	不，非	digestible
infra-	在下	impotence
inter-	中間	dnfrarenal
intra-	在內	intrarenal
iso-	同等	isocoria
-ist	者，家	chemist
-itis	炎	appendicitis
kera-	角	keratitis
leuco-	白	leucoplakia
-lith	石	broncholith
-logist	學家	biologist
-logy	學	biology
-lysis	分解	autolysis
macro-	大	macroscopic
mal-	不良	malpractice
-malacia	軟化	chondromalacia
mega-	巨大	megacolon
mela-	黑	melaena
meso-	中	mesoderm
meta-	變	metabolism

		Example
micro-	小 (微)	micro-organism
mono-	單	monocular
mort-	死	mortality
multi-	多	multiform
-necrosis	壞死	osteonecrosis
neo-	新	neoplasm
neph-, nephro-	腎	nephrotic
neur-, neuro-	神經	neurasthenia
neutro-	中性	neutralization
noct-, nocti-,	夜	nocturia
non-	非	non-infectious
normo-	常規	normoblast
-oid	骨	osteoid
-oma	腫瘤	osteoma
-opia	視力	myopia
-orrhaphy	縫合	herniorrhaphy
os-, oss-, osteo-	骨	ossification
-osis	中毒	acidosis
-otomy	割開，造口術	gastrotomy
paedo-, pedo-	兒童	paediatrics
par-, para-	副，旁	parathyroid
path-, -path	病	psychopath
-penia	缺乏，不足	leucopenia
per-	滲透	perforation
peri-	周圍	pericardium

		Example
-pexy	固定術	gastropexy
phagos-	吞噬	phagocytosis
-philia	好，嗜	basophilia
-phlebo-	靜脈	phlebitis
-phobia	惡／畏	photophobia
-plasty	整形	cystoplasty
-plegia	麻痹	paraplegia
poly-	多	polyphagia
post-	後	postmortem
pro-	前	proerythrocyte
pseudo-	假	pseudocyesis
psycho-	精神	psychogenic
-ptosis	下垂	gastroptosis
pyo-	膿	pyogenic
quadri-, quadru-	四	quadriceps
re-	再	reinfection
rete-, reti-	網	reticular
retro-	後	retropubic
-rhagia	出血	metrorrhagia
-rhoea, -rhea	流，瀉	diarrhoea
sclero-, -sclerosis	硬	arteriosclerosis
-scopy	窺鏡	endoscopy
semi-	半	semilunar
seps-, sept-	毒	septicaemia
-stasis	停，滯	haemostasis

		Example
sub-	下	subcostal
supra-, super-	上	suprapubic
syn-	合	synthesis
-therapy	治療，療法	physiotherapy
-tomy	割開，造口術	tracheostomy
tran-	經	transhepatic
ultra-	超	ultrasound
un-	無，未	undigested
uni-	單	unilateral
-uria, uro-	尿	polyuria
vita-	生命	vitality